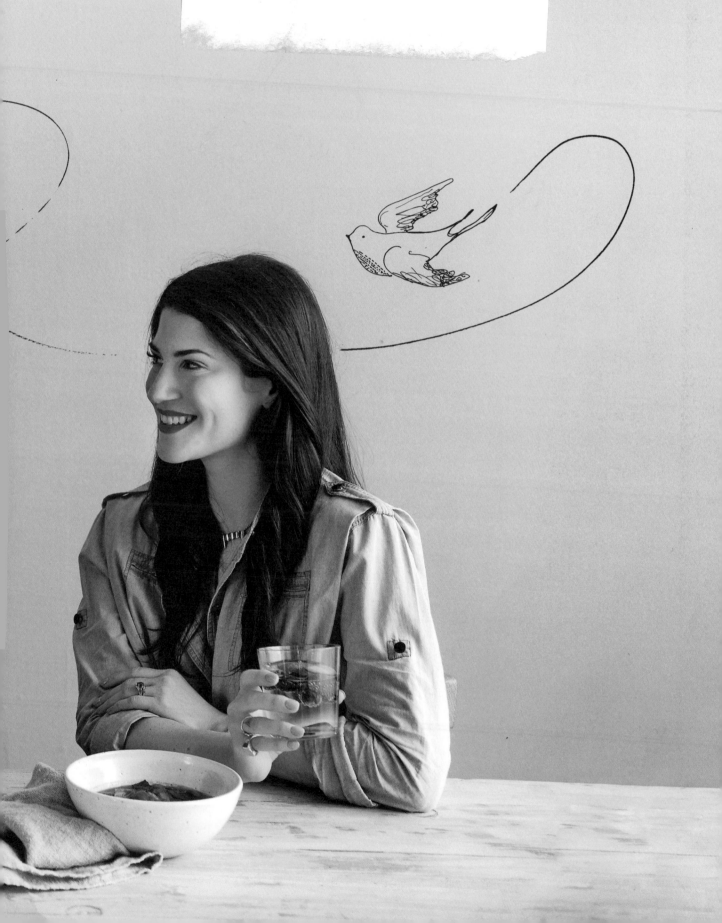

Melbourne born and bred, Tobie Puttock grew up in a family where natural produce was given great precedence, and his appreciation deepened when he went to work for Italian restaurant Caffé e Cucina. He then travelled overseas, honing his skills in restaurant kitchens in Italy, Switzerland and the UK, including time behind the burners at London's River Café and Fifteen London (where he was Jamie Oliver's head chef and right hand man). Tobie then returned home to establish the Australian counterpart, Fifteen Melbourne. Tobie has his own YouTube channel, which is part of Jamie Oliver's Food Tube network. In 2014, he realised a long-held dream by launching Made, a range of restaurant-quality meals that simply need to be warmed up at home, work or wherever you are.
Visit his website at: tobieputtock.com

Georgia Puttock also comes from Melbourne. She spent several years working for some of Australia's premier fashion labels and as a freelance makeup artist before meeting her husband Tobie and moving to London, where she worked at Fifteen London for several years. Her passion for animals led her to study veterinary nursing and she now works as a feline vet nurse at a veterinary clinic in Melbourne. Georgia's food knowledge has been formed by spending years surrounded by Tobie and his local and international chef mates. Her enthusiasm for good-quality fresh produce complements her new interest in health, nutrition and fitness perfectly.

The Chef GETS HEALTHY

TOBIE and GEORGIA PUTTOCK

PHOTOGRAPHY BY SHARYN CAIRNS

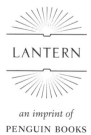

LANTERN

an imprint of
PENGUIN BOOKS

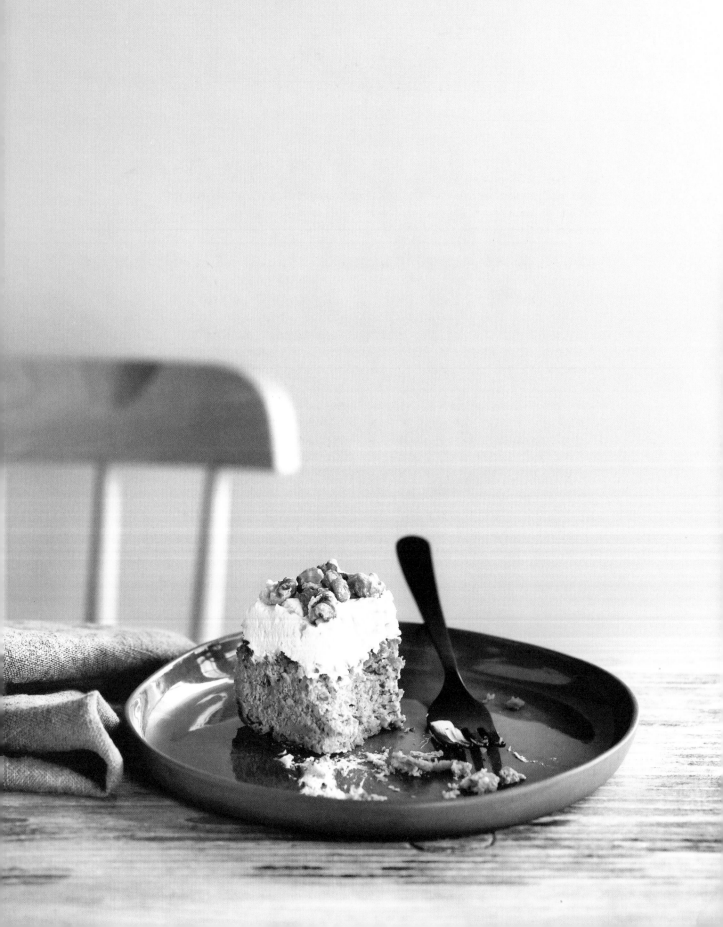

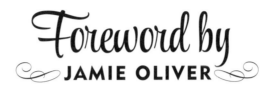

Foreword by
JAMIE OLIVER

When my dear buddy Tobie asked me to write a foreword for this beautiful book he's written with his lovely better half Georgia, my first thought was that this was a potentially dangerous request – having known Tobie for the past 20 years, there are a lot of stories I could share! Luckily for him, I'll keep those to myself for now and focus on the publishable stuff.

So, where do I start? Well, quite simply, Tobie is a funny, straight-talking, honest guy and fantastic cook. Back in the day, we spent a lot of time working and travelling around Italy together, then working at The River Café in London. Tobie then went on to give four amazing years of dedication helping transform my Fifteen London restaurant from a small idea into a huge working reality. So I have to say, it's an absolute honour for me to be writing about this book, which represents the next stage of his life in cooking. And what an important stage it is, all about health, wellbeing, energy and, ultimately, being the very best you can be. Tobie and Georgia have produced an army of recipes that are both tasty and nutritious, but importantly don't compromise on flavour or use copious amounts of ingredients. We all need a bit of help in finding brilliant ideas to enjoy the right stuff, and this book is jam-packed with great, simple, midweek recipes that will get you full up on really delicious, honest, healthy food. Embrace it in your weekly routine and I'm sure you'll feel the benefits – I hope you love it as much as I do.

Well done guys, keep up the good work!

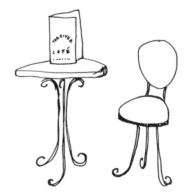

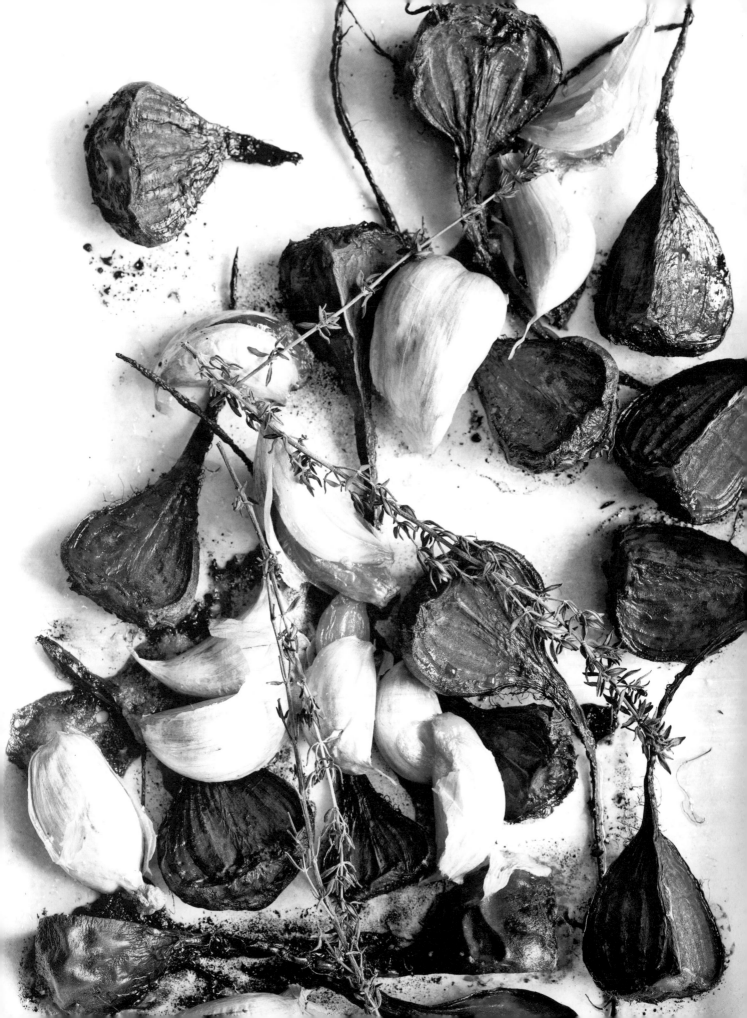

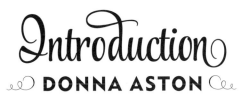

Introduction
DONNA ASTON
NUTRITIONIST/HEALTH & FITNESS EXPERT

I met Tobie through his lovely wife Georgia, who is a client of mine. About eight months after I started working with Georgia, she felt she'd reached a plateau. Tobie prepares their meals (lucky Georgia!) and although he is a fit and active guy, the chef in him was, at that stage, relatively unfamiliar with the concept of kilojoules or moderation. As long as it was a high-quality ingredient, Tobie was liberal with its use. We soon discovered that one of the culprits in Georgia's plateau was lashings of olive oil. Cold-pressed extra virgin, of course! Tobie was surprised to learn that, although it is a healthy ingredient, we don't need copious amounts of it. From this moment on Tobie began taking a keen interest in portion control, balance and moderation. It's no coincidence that in the period straight after Tobie's fine-tuning Georgia blasted through her plateau, reaching her goal body composition and improving her strength and energy levels. Her transformation has been inspiring.

Portion control is another common obstacle for weight loss. Men and women commonly serve themselves equal portions, however a 60-kilo woman doesn't need as much food as a 90-kilo man. As a rule of thumb, the protein portion of a main meal should be about the size of your palm. This is around 80–130 g for women and 160–250 g for men. Fresh plant foods (salads and vegetables) are unlimited – you cannot consume too much colour. Unprocessed fats and oils are necessary for good health, but in moderation. The key to portion control is mindfulness. If you create a relaxed environment that's void of distractions (such as the television and computer) and chew and savour each mouthful, your brain will have time to register that you're full, often before you've finished what's on your plate.

It's clear that Tobie's passion for, and understanding of, food is extraordinary. I'm sure many chefs with his level of experience and expertise would pooh-pooh the idea of trying new techniques or ingredient substitutes, but Tobie has embraced it with gusto. As a nutritionist, my mind automatically gravitates towards the nutritional values, kilojoules and balance of foods, and I have been very impressed with Tobie's innate ability to understand ingredients from all perspectives. In this book he has cleverly combined nutritious, healthy ingredients to create meals that satisfy our nutritional requirements and, importantly, our tastebuds.

Tobie's recipes incorporate whole, fresh ingredients, offering a practical way to help you sustain a healthy weight without feeling like you're missing out. He has been ingenious in his modifications, using herbs and spices to bring flavour and health-promoting properties to savoury dishes, and yoghurt in place of heavier creams to help keep kilojoules at bay. The fact that the recipes are gluten-free makes this book also appropriate for coeliacs and those with a gluten intolerance. Of course, there are a few 'treats' in some of the recipes and desserts, however these are not everyday foods. Georgia is living proof that these tweaks to Tobie's cooking style can have a significant and positive impact on health, fat loss and general wellbeing. Eat and enjoy!

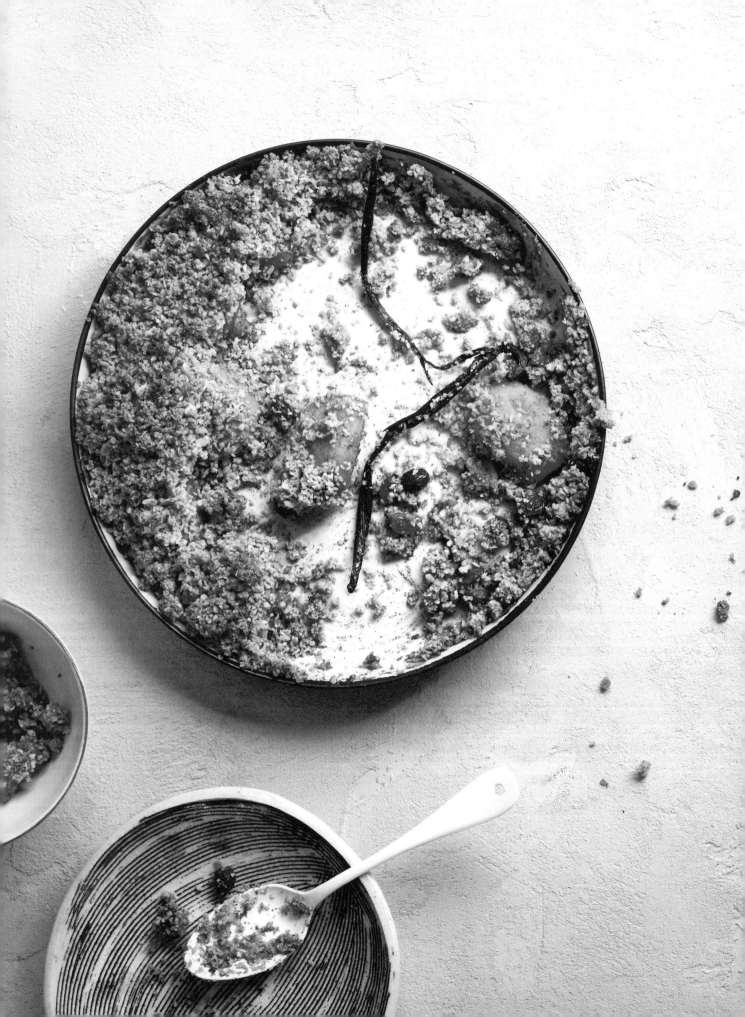

Contents

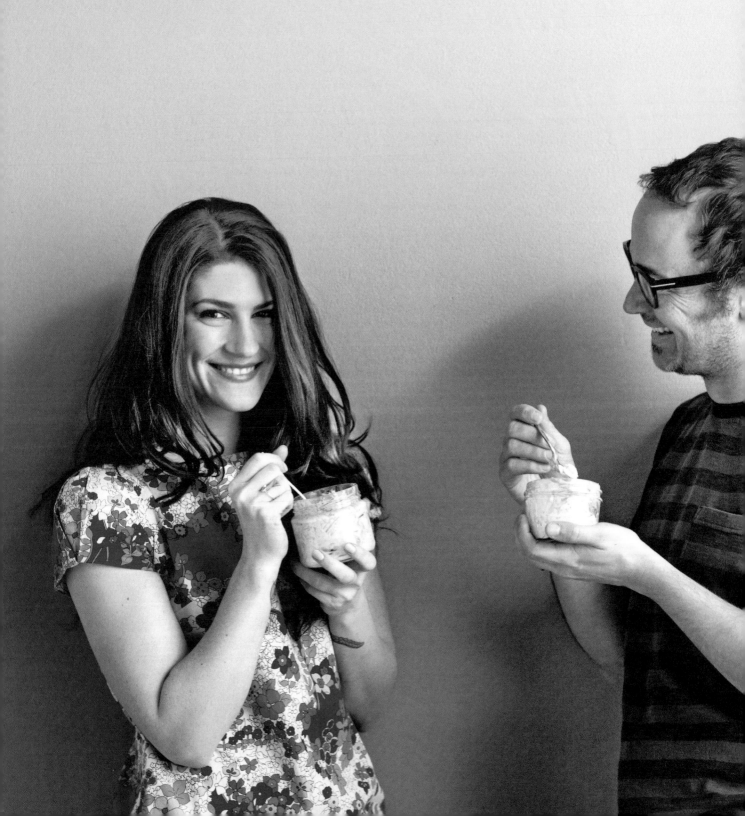

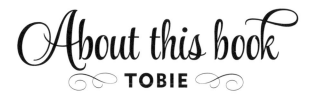

About this book
TOBIE

Traditionally, I would start the introduction to a cookbook like this: 'For many years I travelled the world, working in some of the finest kitchens, eating truffles and walking naked through the hills of Tuscany, yada yada yada.' But the truth is, I started cooking to fund a passion for snowboarding (this hobby costs a lot of money!). What's also true, however, is that cooking has allowed me to travel the world and work in some amazing kitchens in Italy, Switzerland and London.

It was during a brief stint back in Melbourne working at a friend's creperie, AIX Cafe Creperie Salon, that I met Georgia, who's now my wife. For a long time we lived a pretty carefree existence. We travelled the world, working in fantastic restaurants and eating whatever we wanted. Until one day we looked down, then up and down again, and it was clear that the indulgent life of hospitality was catching up with us. I could almost see the lardo, lescure butter, buttermilk ice-cream, deep-fried croquettes, pizza, sourdough, beers . . . you get the picture.

When we moved back to Melbourne, Georgia joined a gym. I think she saw a personal trainer there once a week. I was working at Fifteen Melbourne and Georgia would come in a few nights a week to eat, read and have a glass or three of bubbly while waiting for me to finish up. On my night off, the last thing I wanted to do was cook so we'd always get a big take-away pizza and kick back on the couch with a quenching beer to wash down all that dough.

After some time Georgia realised her training wasn't paying off. Looking back on this now, it's kind of heartbreaking – here was a girl wanting the figure she had when she was nineteen and trying really hard to get the result she wanted. Little did we know I was a large part of the reason she wasn't succeeding. She would come home with books written by nutritionists, but although they may have provided the results she was after, the recipes looked pretty boring to me.

Finally, Georgia visited a training studio in Melbourne owned and run by the talented Donna Aston, and after only a few visits there was positivity in the air. She arranged for me to meet Donna and talk about what I cook at home and while I wasn't over the moon about it, I didn't really think I had anything to worry about; after all, I've been cooking the ultimate Mediterranean diet for years.

When I started talking to Donna (and, more importantly, listening to myself), I soon realised that what we had been eating was far from a healthy Mediterranean diet and more like a restaurant menu. Pretty much every meal of the week was like this, except perhaps breakfast when Georgia would have muesli and I would have coffee. We were simply eating whatever we felt like – thinking about food in terms of flavour and convenience, without considering nutrition at all.

Change had to be made. Georgia was desperate for it and needed me to jump on board 100 per cent. Donna gave me a list of foods we shouldn't eat in abundance and surprise, surprise, they were all things I used in abundance on a day-to-day basis. The main offenders were butter, oils, cheese, bread, pasta, cream and chocolate. And that's just the start of it. Remember, I am a chef and I get paid to make things taste good – all of the above taste good, really good!

Now, for the million-dollar question. Could I create accessible recipes that don't read like a science experiment, with no additives or refined sugar, minimal saturated fats, hardly any refined carbs, lots of proteins and most, *most* importantly, that satisfy my inner chef, both from a cooking point of view and, of course, taste?

The answer is yes, and the proof is in these pages. I will admit that in the beginning my repertoire was small, but when I changed my mindset from 'what I can't cook with' to 'what I can cook with', it became easier. In fact, once I got my head around it, this book quickly became my favourite to write. Gone were the rules of classic Italian cuisine – I began experimenting with flavour combinations I hadn't tried before, adding a pinch of this and handful of that, experimenting with spices I had rarely used and I've gotta tell you, it's been a super-creative experience. I have enjoyed every moment, and according to our friends who have sampled the dishes the old saying 'I can't believe it's not butter!' really describes this style of eating. Big flavours and wholesome ingredients that leave you feeling satisfied, while being good for you at the same time.

The recipes in this book are also gluten-free. For a long time Georgia suffered from IBS and it really controlled her life. When she went to see a nutritionist about it they discovered that one of her triggers was foods containing wheat (and therefore gluten), such as pizza, bread and pasta. She made some adjustments to her diet and now has the IBS well and truly under control. So when we started writing a book of healthy recipes containing nourishing foods, we felt it best to leave gluten out, too.

I would hate to call this book a 'diet book', because that would categorise it. For me, this is just the kind of food we should eat – all the ingredients are natural, there are minimal processed foods, and we use healthy cooking methods like braising, grilling and roasting, with minimal oils. There's an abundance of greens and hardly any carbs, but the really good news is that the flavours are massive.

After I saw Donna and we made all these healthy changes to our diet, my body began to jump on board – I had much more energy and felt awesome. So I started to make some other lifestyle changes to go with my newfound way of eating. For many years while working as a chef, there was a lot of daily pressure and stress. I was always tired, I got headaches all the time and I was generally not that happy. The final straw came when I had a car accident and had to see an optometrist to check my eyesight. He told me I'd lost 35 per cent of vision in my left eye. I was referred to a specialist, who said I had an eye disease called central serous chorioretinopathy, which has been linked to stress and involves a leakage of liquid under the retina. The sad truth was that I wasn't surprised, not one bit. I needed to sort out my stress levels, fast – things needed to change way beyond eating kale. I started running, doing Pilates and also yoga . . . a lot of yoga. Three months later the liquid was almost gone and I was told that my eyes would start self-repairing. In a way, I'm lucky that this condition forced me to take a long hard look at myself.

I generally don't get into the whole 'life quote' thing; I pop them in a basket with mason jars and hip-hop yoga. But there's a snowboarder I follow on Instagram called Kevin Pearce (he has an amazing story, check out *The Crash Reel*, the documentary about it) who listed the non-negotiables in his life and it really stuck with me. I adapted the list to suit my life, but the fundamentals are still the same. When I am disciplined about making time for these rules, I find everything else falls into place easily and I am a better person, inside and out. That's a good thing, right?

Make space for this:

✗ Start the day with exercise.

✗ Do yoga or meditate (even just 5 minutes): morning, noon and night.

✗ Eat a healthy breakfast, lunch and dinner.

✗ Prepare food in advance so there's no excuse to eat crap.

✗ Drink lots of water, at least 2 litres a day.

✗ Get outside, look around (not down at your screen) and listen.

✗ Be present!

✗ Take care of hygiene.

✗ Read and learn something new every day.

✗ Keep in touch with friends and family.

✗ Lead with your heart and keep your mind close behind.

✗ Remember that conscious breathing will always centre you.

✗ Be appreciative and be patient.

✗ Surround yourself with awesome, like-minded people.

✗ Sleep and rest, as much as you feel you need.

Look at this list every day, please, and incorporate as much of it as you can. I know, I know, life is busy and we're all pedalling fast just to keep up, but making time to do the things on this list as often as possible has made a huge difference to my life and I'm sure it will yours.

I sincerely hope you enjoy the recipes I have written with inspiration from my Georgia. We had such a great time working on this book and an even better time recipe testing.

Tobie xx

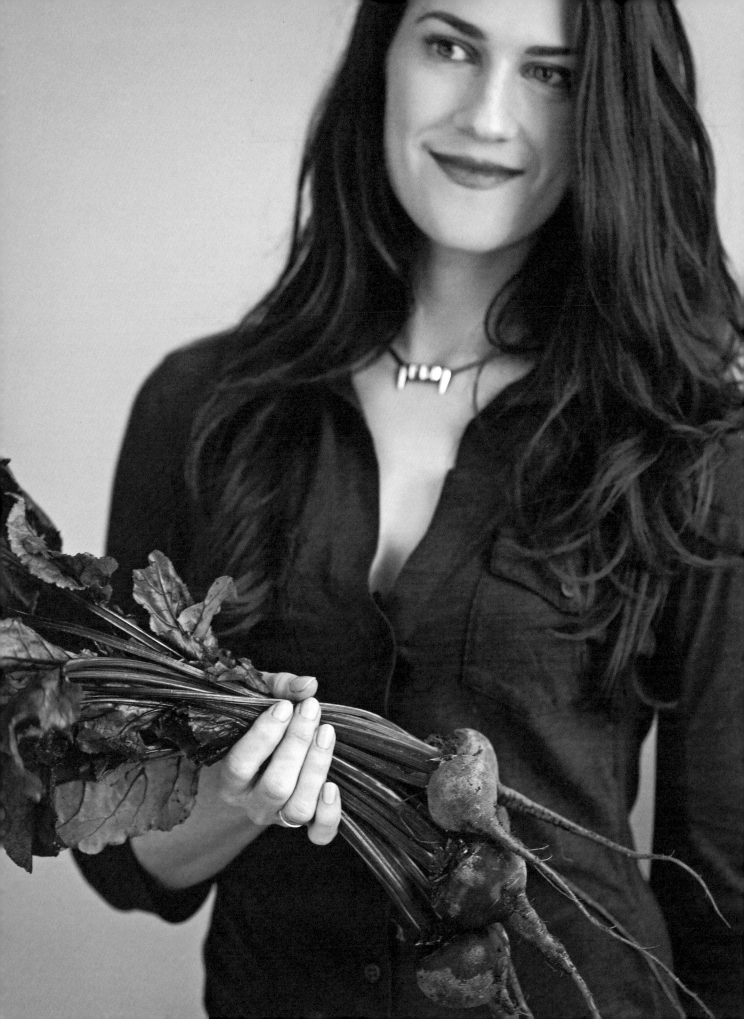

How we eat now
GEORGIA

Weight is a tricky, contentious issue. It is constantly in the media, with celebrities being criticised for being too thin or too fat, while all around the world people in developed nations grow larger and larger. This is due to many factors: convenience, economics, portion size, the list is long. And there is no magical cure for being overweight. Not for a lack of trying either, which is evident in the size and scale of the weight loss industry. But truth be told, there is only one real way to be fit and trim and lose weight: eat a healthy diet and exercise regularly. It may sound boring, but it doesn't have to be! This is a cookbook, not a diet book, with the added bonus of being exceptionally healthy. You do not have to sacrifice flavour to eat a clean, lean diet, though I admit this was a novel concept to Tobie and me initially.

This book came about because in 2001, I met a gorgeous chef in a laneway restaurant in Melbourne. I was working for a fashion boutique close by and after casually eating my lunch there for two weeks on and off, he finally asked me out and the rest is history. Every day, from our first date on, I would go to him at lunch time and he would whip me up a delicious risotto. One month later, my work uniform did not fit. I was a whole size bigger and couldn't figure out why. Tobie suggested the half a block of butter he put in each risotto probably wasn't helping and I was astounded. Those lovely vegetable-filled risottos were bad for me? I had no concept of what sort of foods were weight gainers, aside from the obvious fast food and chocolate. I stopped eating the risottos and started exercising here and there, but nothing much changed and I felt pretty miserable about it.

Ten years later, on a friend's recommendation, I went to see fitness and nutrition guru Donna Aston. We looked at my body composition, using special scales that identify what percentages of your body are made up of fat, muscle and water. The healthy fat range for women falls somewhere between 20–30 per cent, depending on the individual. I was 32.2 per cent. A bit of a shock really. Donna devised a diet plan and exercise regime for me, and gave me the tools to make the necessary lifestyle changes to become the fit and healthy person I am today. Eight months later, I was down to 25 per cent body fat, but I had hit a plateau. Breakfast, lunch and snacks were easy for me to prepare as long as I was organised, but Tobie was still in charge of dinner and Donna felt this was what was holding my progress back. I brought Tobie in to see Donna and she enlightened him on some aspects of nutrition he was unaware of, such as the kilojoule count of extra virgin olive oil.

As a chef, Tobie's job is to make things taste delicious, so removing a lot of his favourite ingredients was challenging, but he's done a brilliant job bringing amazing flavour to the recipes in this book. So, how do we eat now? This book sums it up . . .

Breakfast

I love breakfast. I just can't understand people who don't eat it. It's such an important start to the day, as clichéd as that sounds! Think about it though, your last meal was around 8 to 10 hours ago. You need some premium fuel to get your body working at its optimal level and get that metabolism going. Skip a good brekky and you'll find that around 11 a.m. you'll be getting a bit hungry and as a result you'll make poor nutritional choices, grabbing whatever is closest and easiest, which will generally be something full of sugar, refined carbohydrates, saturated fat and kilojoules. Even eating a commercial product that's labelled as 'healthy', such as commercially made, processed cereals, muffins or muesli bars can send your blood sugar skyrocketing, then plummeting like a rollercoaster leaving you feeling not quite right and hungry for more.

So, what are good options? Fresh produce, low-fat unsweetened yoghurt and small servings of homemade muesli are all good. I'm sorry to say that bread is a 'no' though. I gave it up as it made me bloated and uncomfortable, but it was a good move nutritionally, too. Most bread is high in refined carbohydrates and sodium, and is generally consumed at the expense of fresh plant foods. Refined flour (or carbs) is released quickly during digestion, which further contributes to that whole blood-glucose rollercoaster I mentioned earlier. I won't lie – it was a really hard one to give up, but after about two months I stopped thinking about it and my body is better off without it.

Eggs, on the other hand, are a big 'yes'! They're the most perfect food that exists in nature and you can make so many delicious things with them. One egg contains 6 grams of high-quality protein and all nine essential amino acids. If you are really serious about slimming down, you can leave out some of the yolks as 99 per cent of the fat in an egg is found in the yolk, but if you're pescetarian like me you'll benefit from the extra iron the yolks contain. We use eggs from happy, free-range, cage-free hens.

Soups

Tobie and I eat a lot of soup, all year round. Aside from being totally yummy, we love the fact that you can make a big batch, then freeze single portions for future lunches and dinners. It means you're never caught short and tempted to grab takeaway. Being organised is the key to healthy eating.

Meat

I don't eat meat, but we wanted to include a chapter with the healthy meat recipes that Tobie cooks for himself and our meat-eating friends and family. I don't avoid meat for dietary reasons, but for my own ethics as an animal lover. Lean meat is a valuable source of protein and a good component of a low-carbohydrate diet. It is always best to choose grass-fed meat and understand its provenance.

Fish

Fish has become a staple in my diet since I stopped eating red meat, poultry and pork. It's easy to digest, high in protein and contains omega-3 fatty acids that are necessary for a healthy cardiovascular and nervous system. It also tastes delicious! Make sure you buy sustainable species (see sustainableseafood.org.au for details).

Vegetables and Salads

Vegetables are my new best friends. For a long, long time I didn't really eat them much; even when I became pescetarian I ate mostly bread, pasta and rice dishes instead of increasing my vegetable intake. As a result, I gained weight. But I'm a huge convert now. Vegetables have so much flavour and I've found that the more I eat them, the more I want them. There's nothing I enjoy more now than a brightly coloured salad that's loaded with flavour and texture. You can eat a lot of veggies and really fill up without adding a significant amount of kilojoules to your meal (as long as you're not adding commercially made dressings or lashings of olive oil). All of the vegetable and salad dishes in this book are weeknight staples for us. Served with baked fish or a lean cut of meat, they're really satisfying without leaving you in that state of feeling horribly bloated and over-full.

Desserts

I haven't given up desserts for good, but I only indulge occasionally. I make sure that I really savour each mouthful (no more mindless gobbling!), because when I do this I'm totally satisfied with small portions.

I've always been interested in food, but I used to focus only on flavour and texture. Now, I know so much more about the nutritional side of things and it's been an amazing journey. Some of the most important lessons I've learnt are:

- Be organised. I spend half an hour twice a week chopping veggies for lunch salads.

- Buy a nice water bottle and take it everywhere. You will drink more water!

- Drink green tea. It's really good for you and helps your metabolism.

- Don't drink soft drinks ever. They are FULL of sugar and zero nutrients.

- Cut down your alcohol intake. I've traded wine for low-kilojoule vodka and mineral water with lime juice, and on alcohol-free nights I have mineral water and berries.

- Equip yourself with healthy snacks, such as nuts, a little cheese, fruit and veggies.

- Have an indulgent food once a week, so there's something to look forward to.

- Fresh, unpackaged, unprocessed foods are best. Products labelled as 'low fat' are almost always high in sugar and carbs.

- When eating out, stick to meals with protein and veggies and don't eat the bread!

- Find an exercise that's fun – group sport, dancing, boxing, whatever floats your boat. Aim to walk for 30 minutes every day as well.

- If you start to plateau, keep a food diary to see what you're really eating.

- See a nutritionist if you're really serious about losing weight.

Use this book as a guide to healthy eating (and throw in some moderate exercise), and I'm sure you will notice a difference to your body, and you'll feel great, too. Bon appétit!

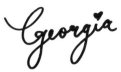

Georgia

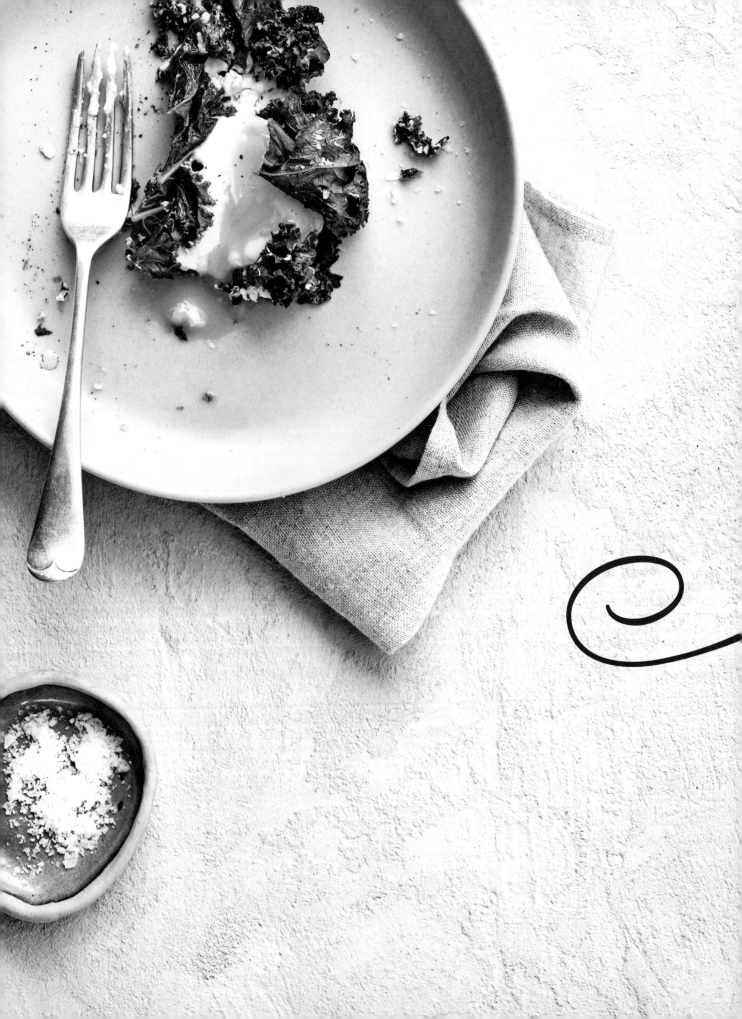

Breakfast

BAKED EGGS *with* CAPSICUM *and* TOMATOES

SERVES: 4

	PER SERVE
ENERGY (KJ/CAL)	567/136
PROTEIN (G)	8
FAT (G)	9
SATURATED FAT (G)	2.5
CARBOHYDRATE (G)	4

1 tablespoon extra virgin olive oil

1 small red onion, thinly sliced

1 red capsicum (pepper), quartered, seeds and membrane removed, cut into thin strips

400 g cherry tomatoes
(I like to use a mixture of varieties)

1 large clove garlic, finely chopped

1 red bird's-eye chilli, finely chopped (optional)

4 eggs

handful of flat-leaf parsley leaves, shredded

sea salt and cracked black pepper

freshly grated parmesan, to serve (optional)

TOBIE I look for about three things in a breakfast: it needs to be easy to make without dirtying too many dishes; it needs to be delicious; and I need to be able to move after I eat it. This ticks all those boxes. The egg whites meander out into the tomatoes to almost bind it together, kind of like a frittata. If you're an anchovy fan like me, add some to the pan just before you put it in the oven.

Preheat the oven to 180°C.

Heat the olive oil in a large ovenproof frying pan over medium heat. Add the onion and capsicum and cook, stirring often, for 5 minutes. Add the tomatoes, garlic and chilli, if using, along with ½ cup (125 ml) of water. Stir to combine, then place the pan in the oven and bake for 5–8 minutes or until the capsicum and onion are softened.

Remove the pan from the oven and use a wooden spoon to make 4 little pockets in the vegetable mixture. Crack an egg into each pocket, then bake for a further 5 minutes or until the eggs are set.

Remove from the oven, sprinkle with the parsley and season with salt and pepper, to taste. Serve scattered with a little parmesan, if desired.

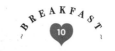

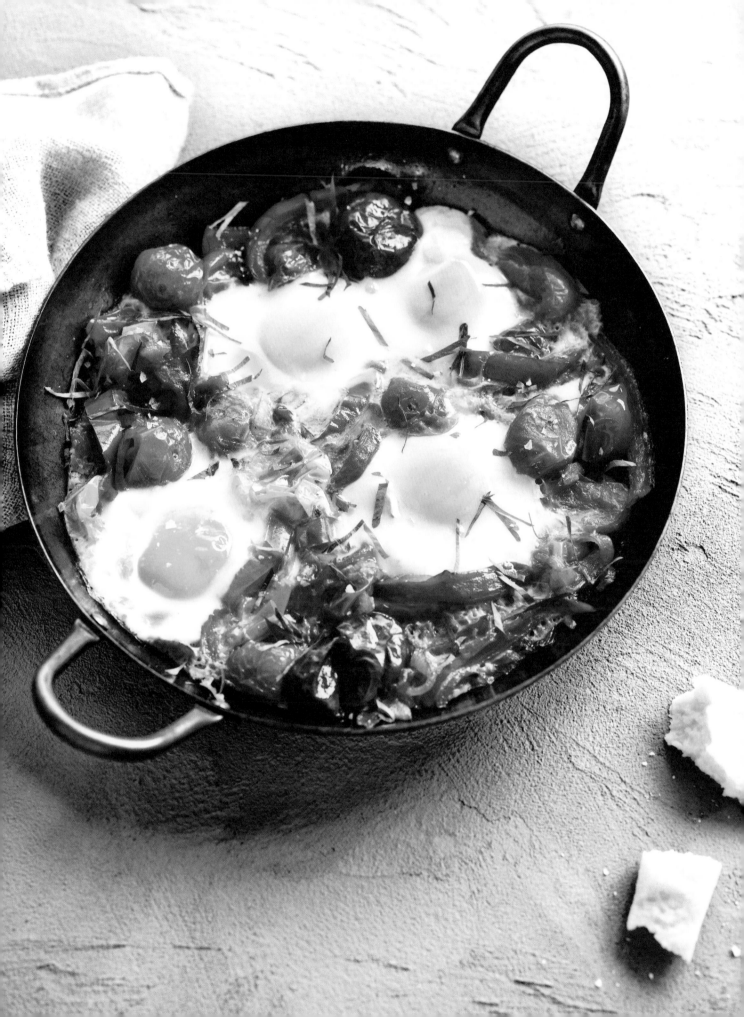

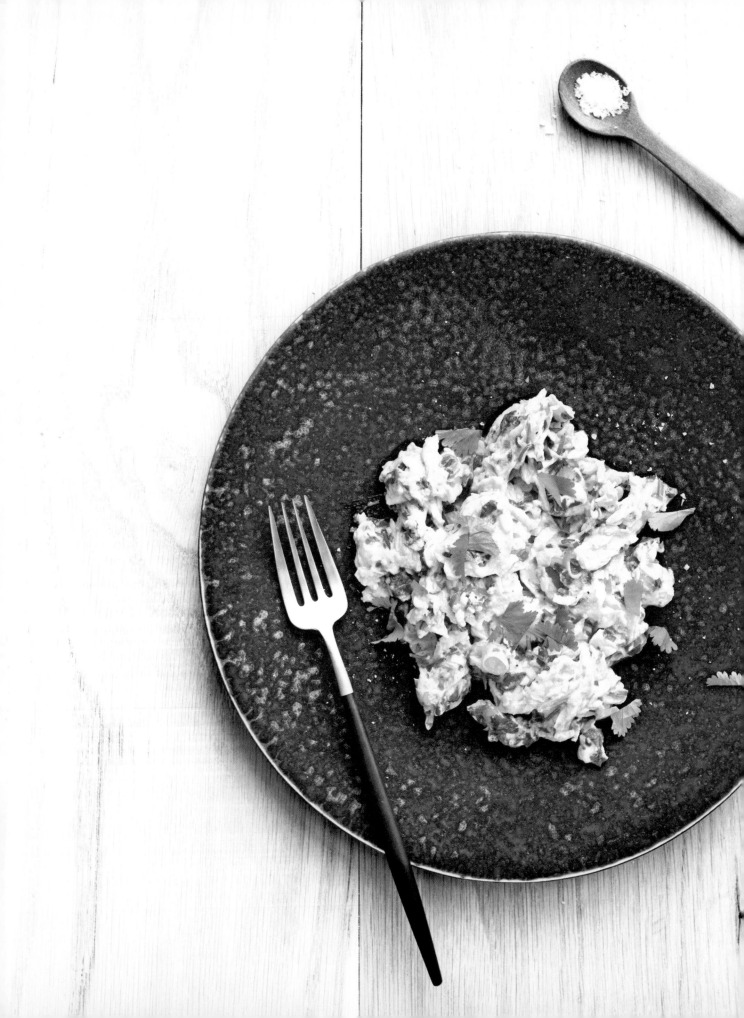

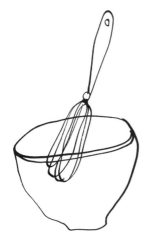

SCRAMBLED EGGS *with* CHILLI, CORIANDER *and* SPRING ONION

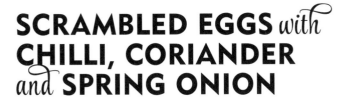

TOBIE I had a version of this at a café in Melbourne and loved it, so I reworked it to suit the requirements of this book and here it is. As Georgia does not eat meat, we have the recipe the way that it's written below. But when I am cooking just for myself I often add a bit of bacon. Before you start cooking the eggs, slice a couple of rashers into batons and cook in the pan, without oil or butter, until browned. Then, melt the butter in the pan, pour the egg mixture over the bacon and continue with the recipe.

GEORGIA I love this healthy take on an old classic – the chilli, coriander and spring onion add loads of flavour.

Crack the eggs into a large bowl and add the milk, coriander, spring onion, chilli, parmesan, if using, and season with a good pinch of both salt and pepper. Use a fork to whisk until everything is combined.

Place a large non-stick frying pan over medium–high heat, add the butter and jiggle the pan around so that the entire base is covered with a film of melted butter. As soon as it is sizzling, add the egg mixture and stir with a wooden spoon. After about 1 minute, remove the pan from the heat and continue to gently stir until the egg has just set. Return to the heat for a moment right before serving if it is too runny for your liking (but remember it becomes rubbery once completely set).

Enjoy as is or serve with rösti, gluten-free bread, grilled shortcut bacon or whatever tickles your fancy.

SERVES: 4

	PER SERVE
ENERGY (KJ/CAL)	645/154
PROTEIN (G)	13
FAT (G)	11
SATURATED FAT (G)	4.5
CARBOHYDRATE (G)	1

8 eggs

2 tablespoons whole-fat milk

2 handfuls of coriander, roughly chopped

2 spring onions, trimmed and thinly sliced

1–2 red bird's-eye chillies, roughly chopped

1 tablespoon freshly grated parmesan (optional)

sea salt and cracked black pepper

2 teaspoons butter

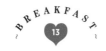

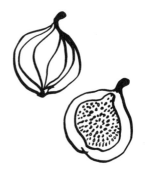

SWEET POTATO BREAD
with CINNAMON RICOTTA *and* FRESH FIGS

Ricotta and cinnamon is a match made in heaven and there's nothing better than smearing it over hot bread. This sweet potato version is pretty light on when it comes to carbs, but has a really beautiful flavour and texture.

This is completely more-ish. I've become addicted to adding cinnamon to sweet dishes, it's a brilliant spice to use when you're forgoing sugar. I use the honey on top sparingly, because even though it's a natural sugar it is not going to help me lose fat by any means. If figs aren't in season, stone fruits and berries are just as yummy.

MAKES: 12 SLICES

	PER SLICE
ENERGY (KJ/CAL)	1126/269
PROTEIN (G)	9
FAT (G)	21
SATURATED FAT (G)	6
CARBOHYDRATE (G)	10

extra virgin olive oil, for greasing

450 g sweet potato, peeled and grated

2½ cups (300 g) almond meal

1 teaspoon bicarbonate of soda

pinch of sea salt

pinch of ground nutmeg

4 eggs, lightly whisked

¼ cup (60 ml) melted virgin coconut oil or extra virgin olive oil

1 teaspoon fresh lemon juice

4 tablespoons fresh ricotta

¼ teaspoon ground cinnamon

4 ripe fresh figs

2 teaspoons honey

Preheat the oven to 160°C. Grease a 24 cm × 13 cm loaf tin using a little olive oil, then line with baking paper and lightly grease the paper. (I am a bit paranoid about things getting stuck, so I grease the paper as well just to be on the safe side, but if you don't want to that's up to you.)

Put the sweet potato in a large bowl. Add the almond meal, bicarbonate of soda, salt and nutmeg and mix until well combined. Mix in the egg, coconut or olive oil and lemon juice. Spoon the mixture into the prepared tin and spread evenly. Bake for 1½ hours or until a skewer inserted into the centre of the loaf comes out clean. If the top of the loaf starts to brown too much during cooking, cover it loosely with foil. Transfer to a wire rack and leave for 20 minutes before removing from the tin.

To serve, cut into thick slices and toast under a grill or in a toaster or sandwich press.

Combine the ricotta and cinnamon, then spread over the hot bread. Tear the figs over the top, drizzle with honey and tuck in.

TIP The bread will keep for up to 5 days in an airtight container, or can be wrapped in plastic film and frozen for up to 2 months.

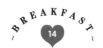

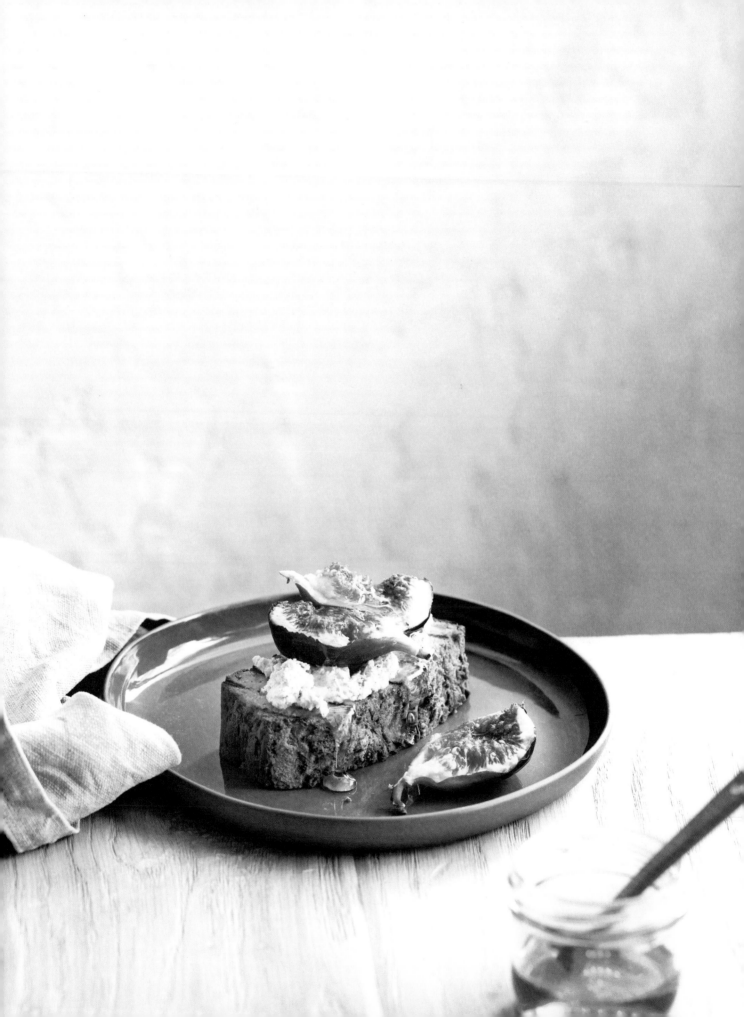

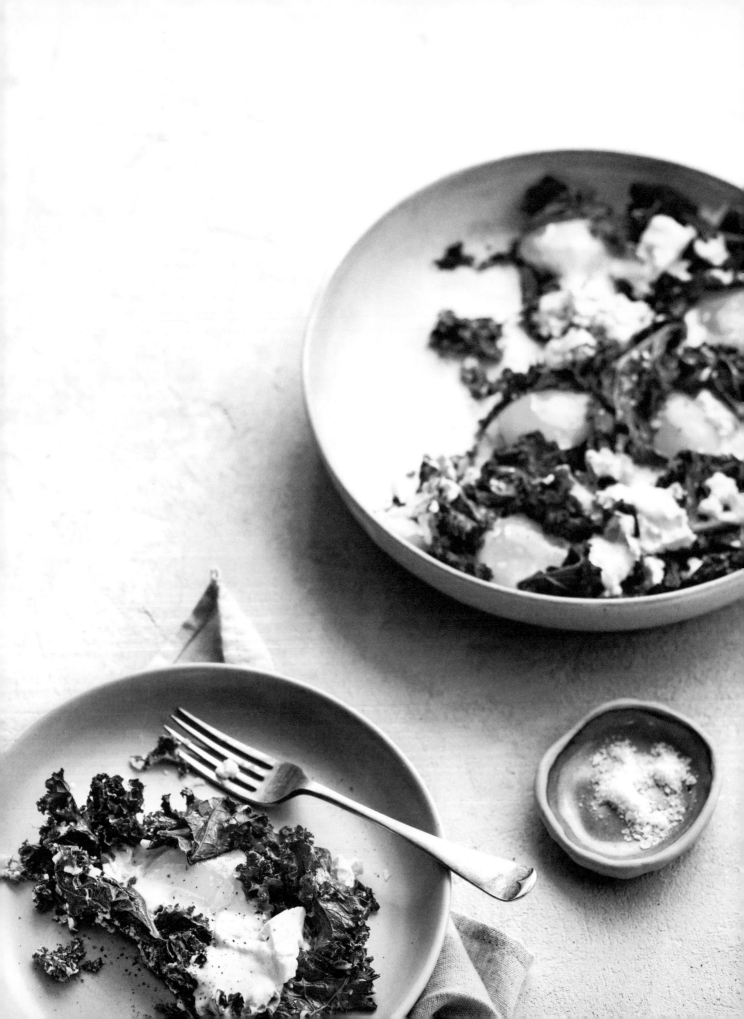

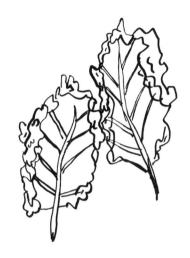

KALE *with* BAKED EGGS, CHILLI *and* FETA

You have got to try this – it's become our go-to weekend breakfast. If you want less heat, remove the seeds from the chilli. I usually pop the whole pan on the table with a spatula and serve it family-style (make sure you warn everyone that the pan is hot), but you can serve individual portions if you prefer.

GEORGIA I can't get enough of kale, it's so versatile and delicious, and really good for you. This is a great way to have it, and the flavour and crunch work really well with the eggs and feta.

Preheat the oven to 180°C.

Heat the olive oil in a large ovenproof non-stick frying pan over medium heat. Add the kale and saute for 1 minute, until slightly wilted. Add the garlic and chilli, season with salt and pepper and cook, stirring, for another minute.

Remove the pan from the heat, make 8 little pockets in the kale mixture and crack an egg into each. Place the pan in the oven and bake for 2 minutes.

Meanwhile, combine the yoghurt and cayenne pepper in a small bowl.

Remove the pan from the oven. Crumble the feta over the kale and eggs, then drizzle with the cayenne yoghurt and return to the oven for a further 3 minutes or until the eggs are set.

Remove from the oven – the egg whites should have run through the kale and set the whole dish almost like a frittata. Serve right away.

SERVES: 4

	PER SERVE
ENERGY (KJ/CAL)	1078/258
PROTEIN (G)	19
FAT (G)	17
SATURATED FAT (G)	6
CARBOHYDRATE (G)	2

1 tablespoon extra virgin olive oil

1 bunch curly kale, stalks trimmed and leaves sliced into 5 cm strips

1 clove garlic, finely chopped

1 red bird's-eye chilli, finely chopped

sea salt and cracked black pepper

8 eggs

100 g low-fat plain Greek-style yoghurt

1 teaspoon cayenne pepper

60 g reduced-fat feta

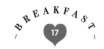

MUSHROOM FRITTATA

This flavour-loaded dish ticks all the health requirements of this book and is one of those great recipes that sets you up for a few days. Having healthy meals that are ready to go makes all the difference when you're busy and don't have the time or energy to cook something from scratch.

As for the mushrooms, you can use whatever type you like. I love to use pine mushrooms when they're in season in autumn, but you will get a delicious result using any mushroom. The art is in the seasoning, so pay attention to your salt and pepper levels.

Preheat the oven to 180°C.

Put the mushrooms in a food processor and pulse briefly until they're finely chopped. (I like to do this as it gives the frittata a lovely texture and great mushroomy colour, but you can simply roughly chop or slice them if you prefer.)

Heat the olive oil and butter in a large, non-stick ovenproof frying pan over medium heat. Add the leek and saute for 5 minutes or until softened. Increase the heat to high, add the mushrooms and cook, stirring often, for 5 minutes or until they are starting to brown.

Meanwhile, use a fork to whisk the eggs, milk, parmesan, parsley, basil and a good pinch of both salt and pepper in a bowl until the egg yolks are all broken.

Add the garlic to the pan, reduce the heat to low and stir to distribute evenly, then pour in the egg mixture. Stir to combine everything, then place the pan in the oven. Bake for 25–30 minutes or until the top of the frittata is set and the centre is slightly firm to the touch. Remove from the oven and set aside to cool for about 10 minutes before cutting into wedges to serve.

SERVES: 6

	PER SERVE
ENERGY (KJ/CAL)	779/186
PROTEIN (G)	14.5
FAT (G)	12.5
SATURATED FAT (G)	4.5
CARBOHYDRATE (G)	3

500 g assorted mushrooms, wiped cleaned with paper towel

1 tablespoon extra virgin olive oil

10 g butter

1 leek, white part only, washed well and thinly sliced

8 eggs

100 ml skim milk

small handful of freshly grated parmesan (about 40 g)

handful of flat-leaf parsley, roughly chopped

handful of basil leaves, roughly torn

sea salt and cracked black pepper

3 cloves garlic, finely chopped

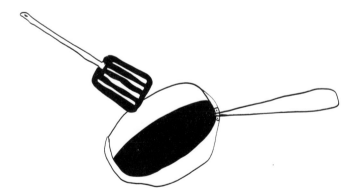

GEORGIA'S MUESLI

GEORGIA Most commercially made mueslis are jam-packed with sugar, which is going to fatten you up and age you. Eek! I make my own variation of a sugar-free muesli recipe given to me by my nutritionist, Donna Aston. As Donna told me, 'sultanas are just little balls of sugar', and this is true of all dried fruit. An important ingredient in this recipe is whey protein isolate powder, which is a great way to incorporate more protein into your breakfast. Protein is an essential nutrient that builds and repairs muscle. It makes you feel fuller, so you're less likely to binge on muffins and cookies in between meals. I eat this muesli most mornings, mixed with a low-fat plain yoghurt and some berries or other fresh fruit on top. Yum!

500 g quinoa flakes
3 cups (250 g) whey protein isolate powder
150 g mixed seeds (such as chia, sunflower, poppy, pepitas, linseeds)
150 g mixed raw unsalted nuts
2 tablespoons desiccated coconut
1 tablespoon ground cinnamon
2 vanilla beans, split lengthways and seeds scraped

Put all the ingredients in a large bowl and mix until really well combined.

Pour the muesli into an airtight container and store in a cool, dark cupboard.

TIP This muesli will keep in an airtight container in a cool, dark place for up to 1 month.

MAKES: ABOUT 1 KG

	PER 50G
ENERGY (KJ/CAL)	911/218
PROTEIN (G)	16
FAT (G)	8.5
SATURATED FAT (G)	1
CARBOHYDRATE (G)	18

CHEAT'S BERRY YOGHURT

TOBIE This makes me think of John Travolta in *Pulp Fiction* talking about the 'little differences'. Mixing some frozen berries and maple syrup into your yoghurt is such a little thing, but it has such a big effect.

GEORGIA I steer clear of commercially made flavoured yoghurts, even the low-fat varieties, because they are generally loaded with sugar. I've always enjoyed the slightly tart flavour of plain Greek-style yoghurt, but mixing in berries makes it even tastier.

¾ cup (200 g) low-fat plain Greek-style yoghurt
250 g frozen mixed berries (you can also use fresh)
1 tablespoon pure maple syrup or honey (optional)

Place the yoghurt, half the berries and the maple syrup or honey, if using, in a food processor and pulse a few times, until smooth.

Add the remaining berries and pulse once or twice, just to break them up a little bit but so there are still chunks of berry in there. Transfer to an airtight container and keep in the fridge.

TIP The yoghurt will keep in an airtight container in the fridge for up to 1 week.

SERVES: 4

	PER SERVE
ENERGY (KJ/CAL)	342/82
PROTEIN (G)	3.5
FAT (G)	1
SATURATED FAT (G)	0.5
CARBOHYDRATE (G)	12.5

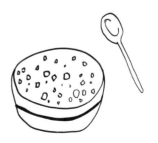

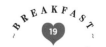

BIRCHER MUESLI POTS

TOBIE It's 6:30 a.m. The alarm goes off and you hit the snooze button, then it goes off again and the rush to get to work begins. A quick shower, then you throw on your clothes and shove down some food. Sound familiar? Eating well is all about being organised – spending a little time when you aren't busy so you have something ready for the rush hour. This sort of thing is perfect. It needs to sit overnight so the muesli becomes beautiful and chewy the next day. If you want to get a bit fancy, you could use the Cheat's berry yoghurt (see page 19) instead of plain yoghurt.

1 small apple, grated

4 tablespoons Georgia's muesli (see page 19)

4 tablespoons low-fat plain Greek-style yoghurt

handful of berries (if using strawberries, hull and halve them)

Combine the apple, muesli and yoghurt in a bowl. Spoon into 2 little jars or takeaway containers, pop on the lids and allow to sit overnight. Serve topped with the berries, or mix them through if you like.

SERVES: 2

	PER SERVE
ENERGY (KJ/CAL)	568/136
PROTEIN (G)	7.5
FAT (G)	3
SATURATED FAT (G)	1
CARBOHYDRATE (G)	18

BANANA and MACADAMIA BUTTER BREAKFAST SMOOTHIE

TOBIE I did the kale smoothie thing for a while, but in the morning I'm really after something that's comforting and is going to give me energy. This smoothie does the trick. You can use any type of homemade nut butter.

2 ripe bananas, peeled

1 cup (250 ml) low-fat or skim milk

1 cup (280 g) low-fat plain Greek-style yoghurt

1 teaspoon honey

1½ tablespoons Homemade macadamia nut butter (see page 190)

good pinch of ground cinnamon

good handful of ice cubes

Put everything in a blender, add ½–1 cup (125–250 ml) of water and blitz until smooth. Too easy!

SERVES: 2

	PER SERVE
ENERGY (KJ/CAL)	1670/400
PROTEIN (G)	15.5
FAT (G)	17.5
SATURATED FAT (G)	4.5
CARBOHYDRATE (G)	42

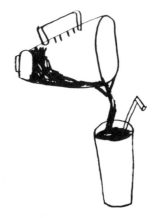

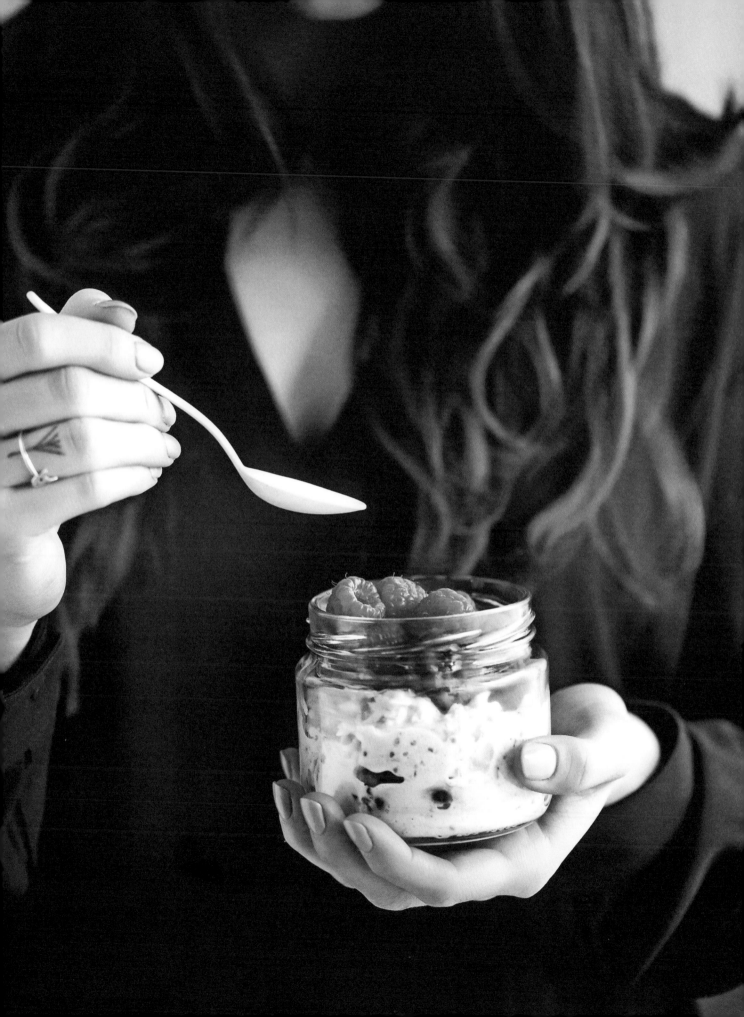

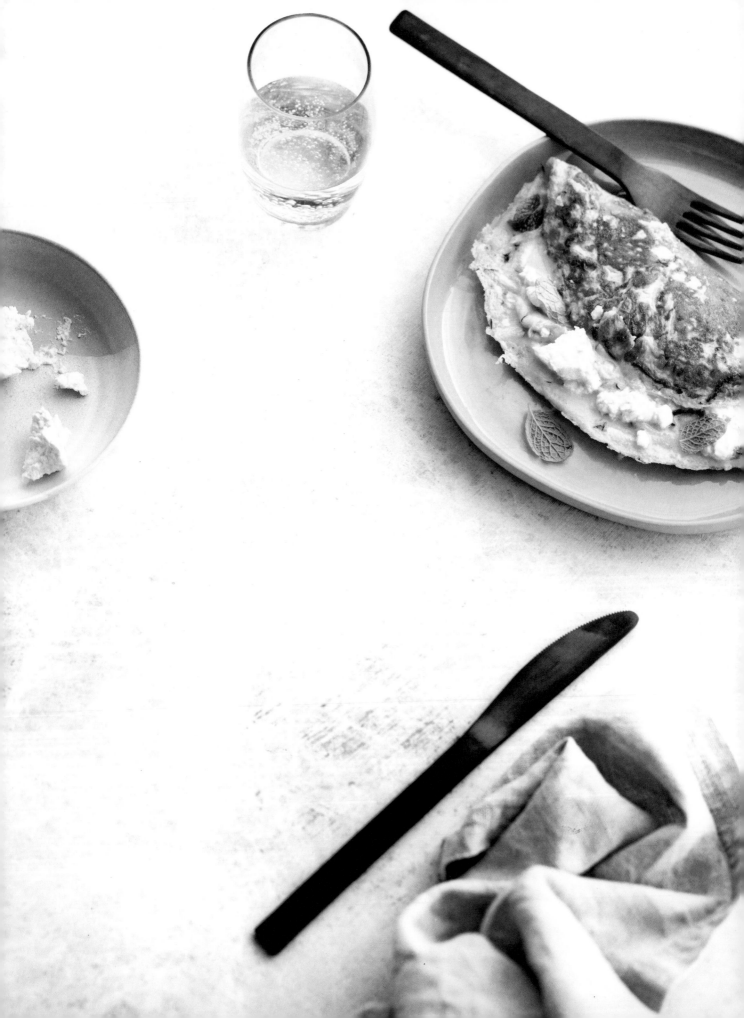

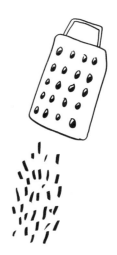

OMELETTE *with* SHREDDED ZUCCHINI, GOAT'S CHEESE *and* MINT

TOBIE This is a great recipe to get you going in the morning and it's super-quick. It normally takes me under 5 minutes to get the first omelette on the plate, but let's be honest, I've made a few in my time! When I make it, one of the first things I do is pop the pan over low heat. This means the pan is hot by the time everything else is ready to go, so I can start cooking right away.

GEORGIA I could eat this for breakfast, lunch or dinner. It's quick, easy and delish, without being high in kilojoules.

Heat a non-stick frying pan, about 30 cm in diameter, over low–medium heat. Crack the eggs into a bowl and add the milk or water and zucchini. Season with a pinch of both salt and pepper and gently whisk with a fork until the egg yolks are broken and the zucchini is mixed in.

Add the butter to the hot frying pan and jiggle the pan so the entire base has a thin film of melted butter over it. Add the egg and zucchini mixture and jiggle the pan so it is evenly distributed. Cook until the egg starts to set at the edges. Crumble the goat's cheese over half the omelette, then scatter over the mint leaves.

Cook until the omelette is set around the edges and the centre is cooked to your liking – I like mine a bit runny in the middle. As soon as it's set enough to flip one side over, it's good for me. Use a spatula to fold the side without the filling over the side with the filling, so you have a half-moon shape. Once the underside is slightly golden, transfer to a serving plate and eat right away.

SERVES: 1

	PER SERVE
ENERGY (KJ/CAL)	771/184
PROTEIN (G)	15
FAT (G)	13
SATURATED FAT (G)	5.5
CARBOHYDRATE (G)	1.5

2 eggs

1 tablespoon whole-fat or skim milk, or water

½ zucchini (courgette), coarsely grated

sea salt and cracked black pepper

½ teaspoon butter, to grease

10 g soft goat's cheese

6 mint leaves, torn if large

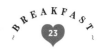

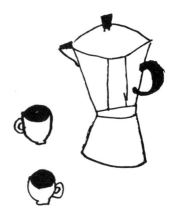

BANANA *and* PECAN BREAD

MAKES: 10 SLICES

	PER SLICE
ENERGY (KJ/CAL)	1236/296
PROTEIN (G)	7.5
FAT (G)	24.5
SATURATED FAT (G)	6
CARBOHYDRATE (G)	10.5

extra virgin olive oil, to grease

300 g ripe bananas (about 2½)

50 g melted virgin coconut oil

2 tablespoons pure maple syrup

1 tablespoon vanilla extract

2 teaspoons ground cinnamon

1 teaspoon bicarbonate of soda

1 teaspoon fresh lemon juice

3 eggs, lightly whisked

200 g almond meal

100 g pecan halves

TOBIE I've always thought of banana bread as a legitimate way to eat cake for breakfast. We don't have it often, but I couldn't bear saying goodbye to it completely, so I took up the challenge of creating a recipe that is low in saturated fat and free of refined sugar and gluten, without tasting like cardboard. I think I nailed it!

GEORGIA I love sweet and savoury breads, and I still eat them, but more as a treat than an everyday kind of thing. This banana bread is awesome, because it's healthy, satisfying and tastes divine.

Preheat the oven to 160°C. Grease a 20 cm × 10 cm loaf tin with a little olive oil, line with baking paper and then grease the paper. (I am a bit paranoid about things getting stuck, so I grease the paper as well just to be on the safe side, but if you don't want to that's up to you.)

Put the banana, coconut oil, maple syrup, vanilla, cinnamon, bicarbonate of soda and lemon juice in a bowl and mash well with a fork. Add the egg, almond meal and pecans and use a wooden spoon to mix until combined.

Spoon the mixture into the prepared tin and spread evenly. Bake for 45 minutes or until a skewer inserted into the centre of the loaf comes out clean. If the top of the loaf starts to brown too much during cooking, cover it loosely with foil. Transfer to a wire rack and leave for 20 minutes before removing from the tin.

Cut into slices and serve warm, at room temperature or toasted.

TIP This will keep for up to 5 days in an airtight container, or can be wrapped in plastic film and frozen for up to 2 months.

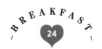

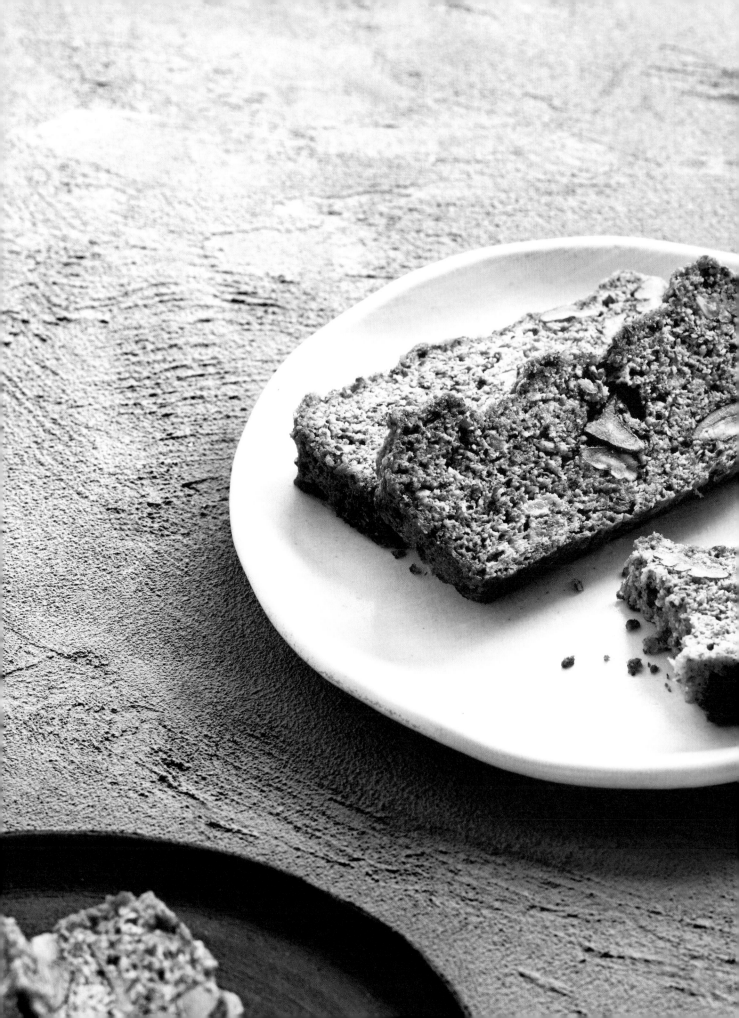

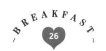

CAULIFLOWER, THYME, MUSTARD and CHEDDAR FRITTATA

SERVES: 6

	PER SERVE
ENERGY (KJ/CAL)	1109/265
PROTEIN (G)	18
FAT (G)	19
SATURATED FAT (G)	9
CARBOHYDRATE (G)	4

600 g cauliflower florets

1 tablespoon extra virgin olive oil

3 teaspoons gluten-free wholegrain mustard

2 teaspoons smoked paprika

8 eggs, lightly whisked

½ cup (125 ml) whole-fat or skim milk

150 g grated good-quality cheddar

handful of flat-leaf parsley leaves

1 red bird's-eye chilli, finely chopped

sea salt and cracked black pepper

½ teaspoon butter

Roast tomato sauce (see page 191), to serve (optional)

TOBIE Frittata must have been one of the first things I learnt to make back in the nineties at Melbourne's Caffé e Cucina. It's the kind of thing I love to make on a Sunday morning.

GEORGIA I adore frittata! Tobie makes it for breakfast and then I take leftovers for lunch for the next 2 days, dressed up with a quarter of an avocado and some dried chilli flakes.

Preheat the oven to 220°C.

Line a baking tray with baking paper. Place the cauliflower florets in a large bowl, add the olive oil and toss to combine. Scatter the florets over the lined tray and bake for 25–30 minutes or until they are quite dark in colour. Remove and set aside to cool. Reduce the oven temperature to 200°C.

Combine the mustard and paprika in a large bowl. While whisking with a fork, slowly pour in the egg and milk, whisking until combined. Add the cauliflower, two-thirds of the cheddar, the parsley, chilli and a good pinch of both salt and pepper. Stir to distribute evenly and break up the cauliflower.

Place a large flameproof and ovenproof non-stick dish (about 30 cm long and 4–5 cm deep) over high heat. Once hot, add the butter and jiggle the pan around so that the entire base is covered with a film of melted butter.

Pour the frittata mixture into the pan and immediately turn off the heat. Use a fork to flatten the surface, then scatter the remaining cheddar over the top. Bake for 15 minutes or until the top of the frittata is set and the centre is slightly firm to the touch.

Remove from the oven and set aside to cool for about 5 minutes before cutting into wedges. Serve with roast tomato sauce alongside, if desired.

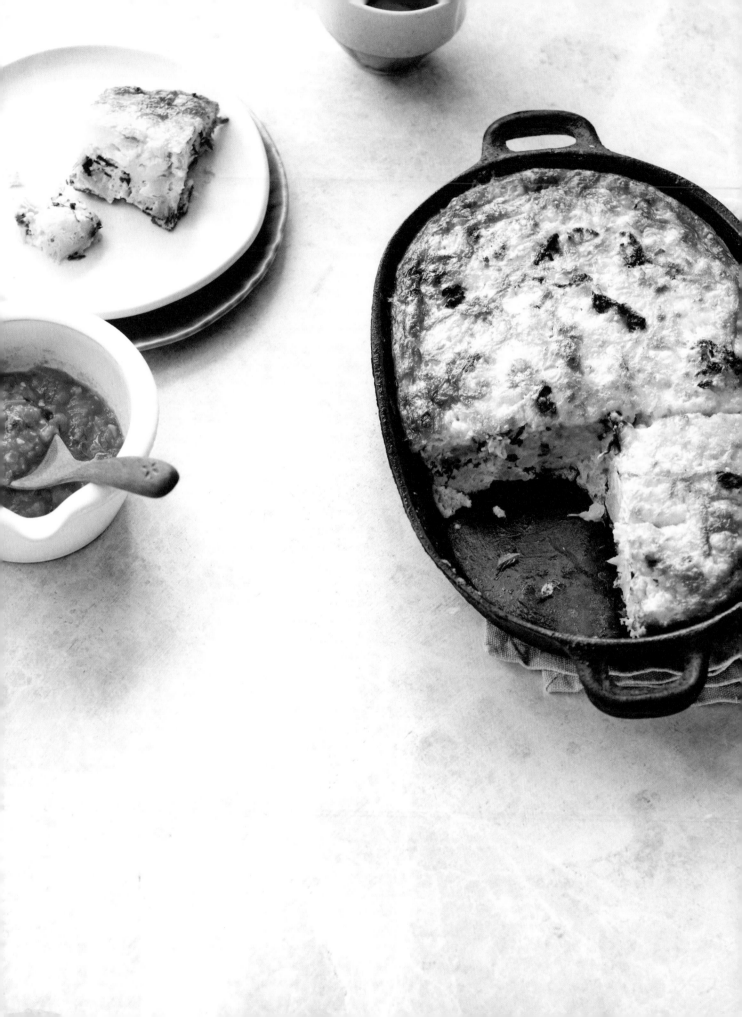

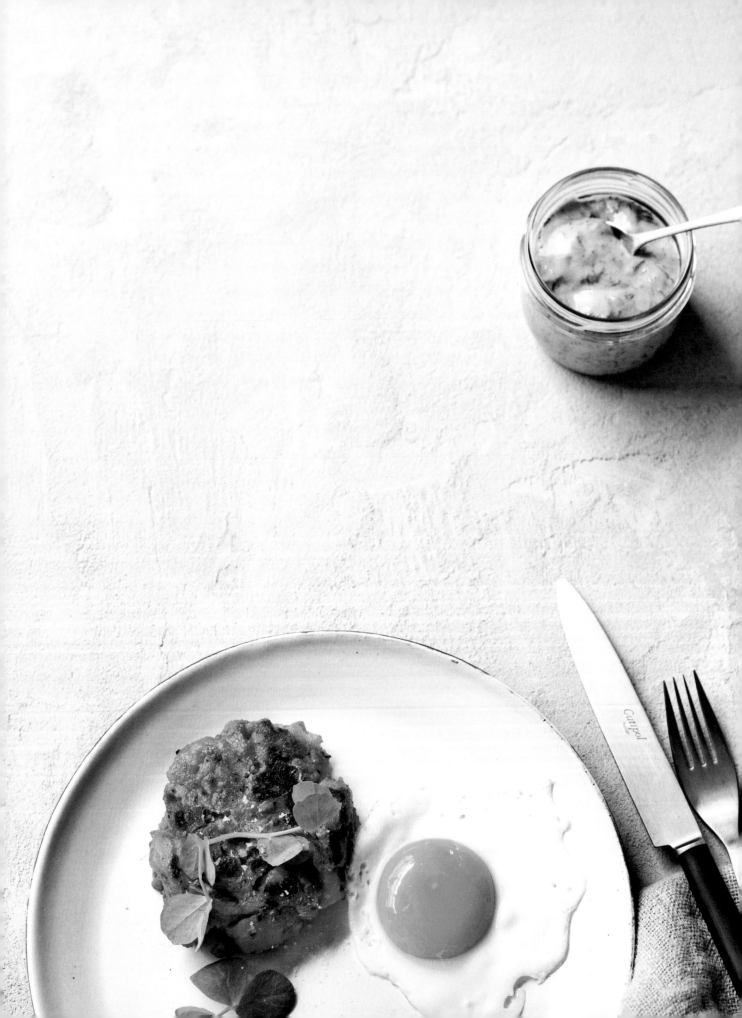

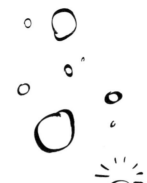

BUBBLE *and* SQUEAK *with* FRIED EGGS *and* DILL SAUCE

TOBIE When I was living in London I remember watching the lovely lady at the local greasy spoon almost ladling butter into a pan before adding the roast veggies to make bubble and squeak. It was delicious, rich and most definitely not a recipe that could go in this book! Instead, here is a version that's hip friendly. I will be honest with you, a tiny bit of butter (about a teaspoon) helps stop the patties sticking to the pan, but I'll leave that decision up to you.

GEORGIA I'd hardly ever eaten bubble and squeak before I met Tobie, but I'm a huge fan now. Whenever we have roast veggies for dinner we cook extra so we can use the leftovers to make this.

Put the roasted vegetables in a bowl and add the parmesan, if using, and a good pinch of both salt and pepper. Mash with a potato masher, then shape into four equal-sized patties.

Heat the oil in a large non-stick frying pan over medium heat. Carefully lower the patties into the pan, then reduce the heat to low–medium and jiggle the pan for the first minute of cooking to help prevent the patties sticking. Cook for 3–4 minutes on each side, until browned all over.

Meanwhile, heat a separate non-stick frying pan over medium heat, then add a teaspoon of olive oil and use paper towel to rub it over the pan to leave a light film. Reduce the heat to low, crack in the eggs and cook until the whites have set, about 2–3 minutes.

Remove the bubble and squeak from the pan and place on paper towel for a moment to drain off any excess oil. Transfer to serving plates and add the fried eggs and some cress or rocket. Season with salt and pepper and serve right away, with the dill sauce alongside.

SERVES: 4

	PER SERVE
ENERGY (KJ/CAL)	1083/259
PROTEIN (G)	9.5
FAT (G)	17.5
SATURATED FAT (G)	3.5
CARBOHYDRATE (G)	13

400 g leftover Roasted root vegetables (see page 117)

1 tablespoon freshly grated parmesan (optional)

sea salt and cracked black pepper

2 tablespoons olive oil, plus extra for greasing

4 eggs

pea cress, picked watercress or rocket, to serve

2 tablespoons Swedish dill sauce (see page 182)

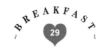

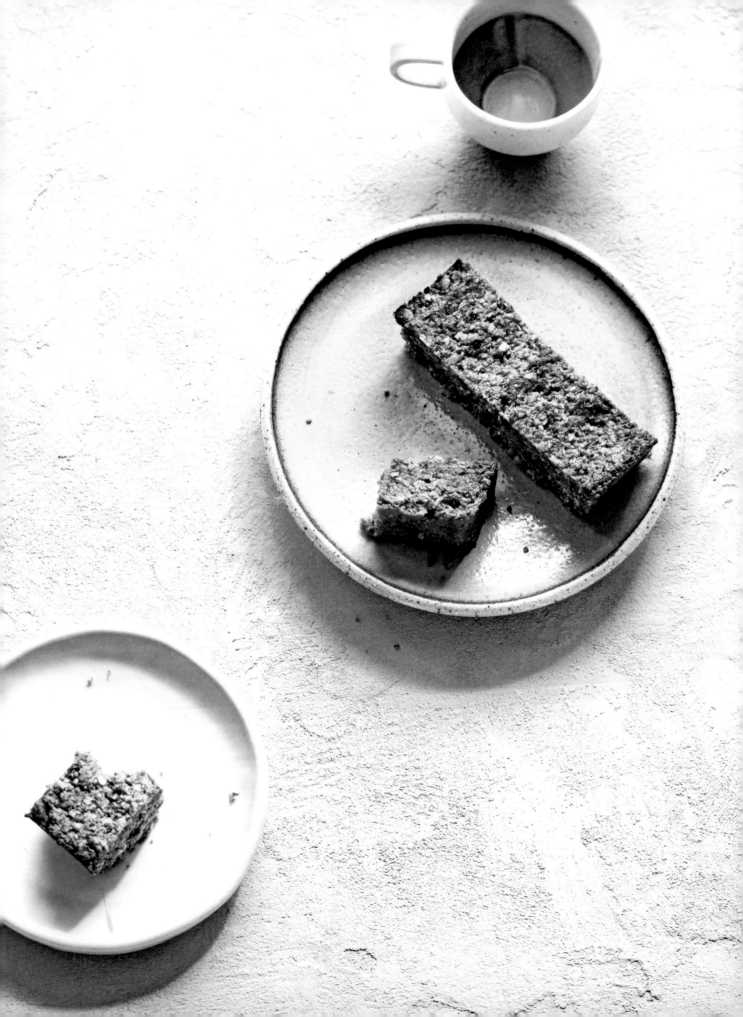

APPLE *and* CINNAMON BREAKFAST BAR

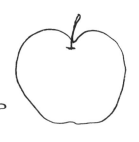

`TOBIE` No matter how busy your mornings might be, if you make this slice on the weekend you'll be set for the week. It's a miracle we have a picture of it to go in the book, because when I made it at the photo shoot the team demolished it in a matter of seconds. It's one of those great recipes that is dead easy to make and doesn't require any fancy ingredients, but comes out beautifully.

`GEORGIA` Tobie loves this for breakfast, but I love it as a snack – if I have a small slice mid-morning it will easily get me through to lunchtime. The walnuts are full of protein, vitamins and minerals.

Preheat the oven to 180°C. Line a baking tray with baking paper.

Scatter the walnuts over the lined tray in a single layer and bake for 7–10 minutes, until fragrant. Remove from the oven and set aside to cool.

Line the base and sides of a 20 cm × 10 cm loaf tin with baking paper. Pop the toasted walnuts, almond meal, quinoa flakes, dates, cinnamon and salt into a food processor and pulse until the mixture resembles coarse breadcrumbs. Add the apple and pulse until the ingredients bind together.

Tip the mixture into the lined tin and use your hands or a spatula to pack it down so it's an even thickness all over (be sure to push it into the edges).

Bake the slice for 20 minutes, then transfer to a wire rack. Leave for 10 minutes before removing from the tin. Cool for 10–20 minutes before cutting into 10 bars.

TIP Store the bars in an airtight container in the fridge for up to 1 week.

MAKES: 10

	PER BAR
ENERGY (KJ/CAL)	1384/331
PROTEIN (G)	7
FAT (G)	21.5
SATURATED FAT (G)	1.5
CARBOHYDRATE (G)	25.5

2 cups (200 g) walnuts

1 cup (120 g) almond meal

1 cup (110 g) quinoa flakes

1½ cups (210 g) pitted dates, halved

2 teaspoons ground cinnamon

good pinch of sea salt

2 granny smith apples, peeled, cored and coarsely grated

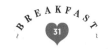

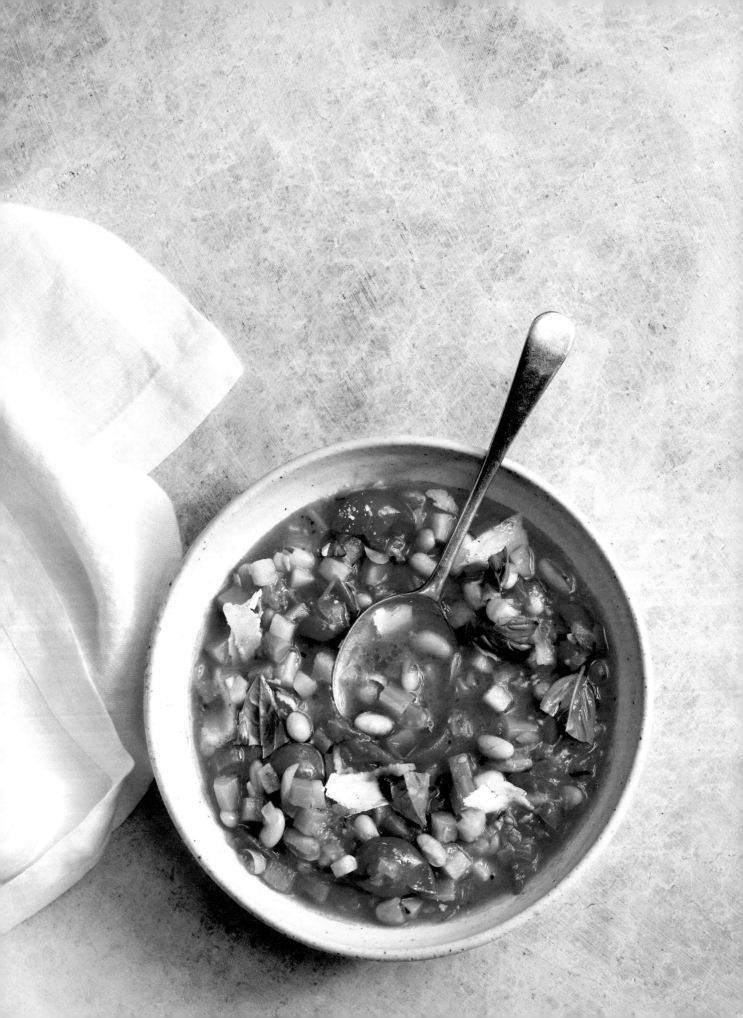

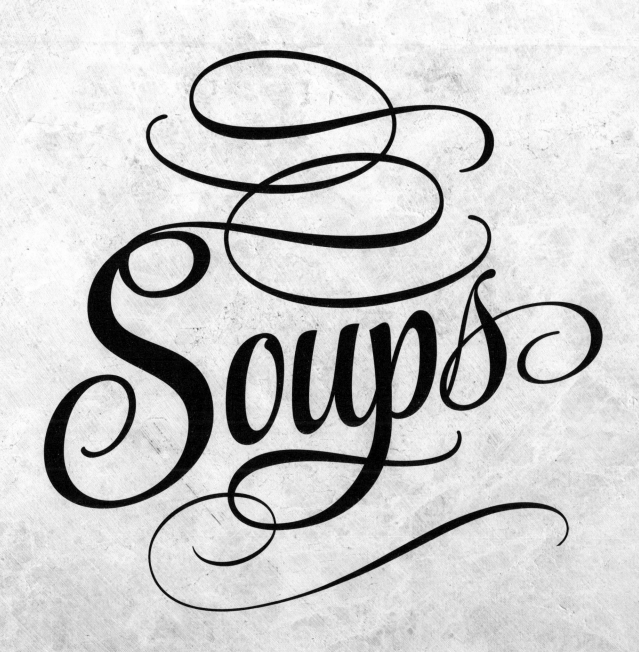

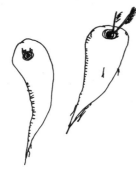

PARSNIP SOUP
with POACHED EGG

SERVES: 6

	PER SERVE
ENERGY (KJ/CAL)	884/211
PROTEIN (G)	9.5
FAT (G)	11
SATURATED FAT (G)	2.5
CARBOHYDRATE (G)	16

2 tablespoons olive oil

1 red onion, roughly chopped

2 stalks celery, trimmed and roughly chopped

1 teaspoon dried chilli flakes (optional)

1 tablespoon thyme leaves

2 bay leaves

4 cloves garlic, roughly chopped

8 medium parsnips, peeled and roughly chopped

2 litres water or gluten-free stock (vegetable or chicken)

sea salt and cracked black pepper

1 teaspoon apple cider vinegar

6 eggs

truffle oil, to serve (optional)

TOBIE Pureed soups normally gain their rich flavour and smooth texture through added fats in the form of cream, butter and excessive olive oil. I have been making this soup for a while now, without any of these added fats, and the beautiful and natural parsnip flavour does all the talking. The poached egg brings a lovely richness and some much-wanted protein. The soup still tastes great without it, but for me it is an essential element.

GEORGIA This is one of my favourite soups to take to work (minus the poached egg, of course). I also pack a vial of black truffle oil and drizzle a tiny bit over the top once it's heated up – the flavours work perfectly together.

Heat the olive oil in a large heavy-based saucepan or stockpot over high heat. Add the onion, celery, chilli flakes, if using, thyme, bay leaves and garlic and cook, stirring often, for 5 minutes. Add the parsnip and cook for a further 5 minutes, stirring from time to time. Add the water or stock and bring to the boil, then reduce the heat and hold at a gentle simmer for 40 minutes or until the parsnip can be pierced easily with a small knife. Remove the bay leaves.

Use a blender, stick blender or food processor to puree the soup until smooth. (If using a food processor or blender, cool the soup slightly before processing and do it in batches.) Taste and adjust the seasoning with salt and pepper as necessary. You can also adjust the consistency by reducing the soup further to thicken it or adding some more stock or water to thin it.

Fill a large saucepan with enough water to just submerge a whole egg, add the vinegar and bring to a simmer over high heat. Crack an egg into a small bowl. Use a spoon to gently move the water around in a circular motion like a whirlpool. Gently lower the egg into the water, then continue to add up to 2 more eggs in the same manner. Turn off the heat and cover the pan with a lid, then set aside for 5 minutes. Use a slotted spoon to transfer each egg to a bowl of cold water. Repeat to poach the remaining eggs. Remove and place on paper towel briefly to drain. Transfer the eggs in the cold water back to the hot water in the pan to heat up again, then drain on paper towel.

Serve the hot soup with a poached egg in the middle, a drizzle of truffle oil, if using, and a grind of pepper.

TIP This soup freezes really well (without the poached eggs and truffle oil) and will keep for up to 2 months. I often make a double batch and then freeze single-serve portions in airtight containers.

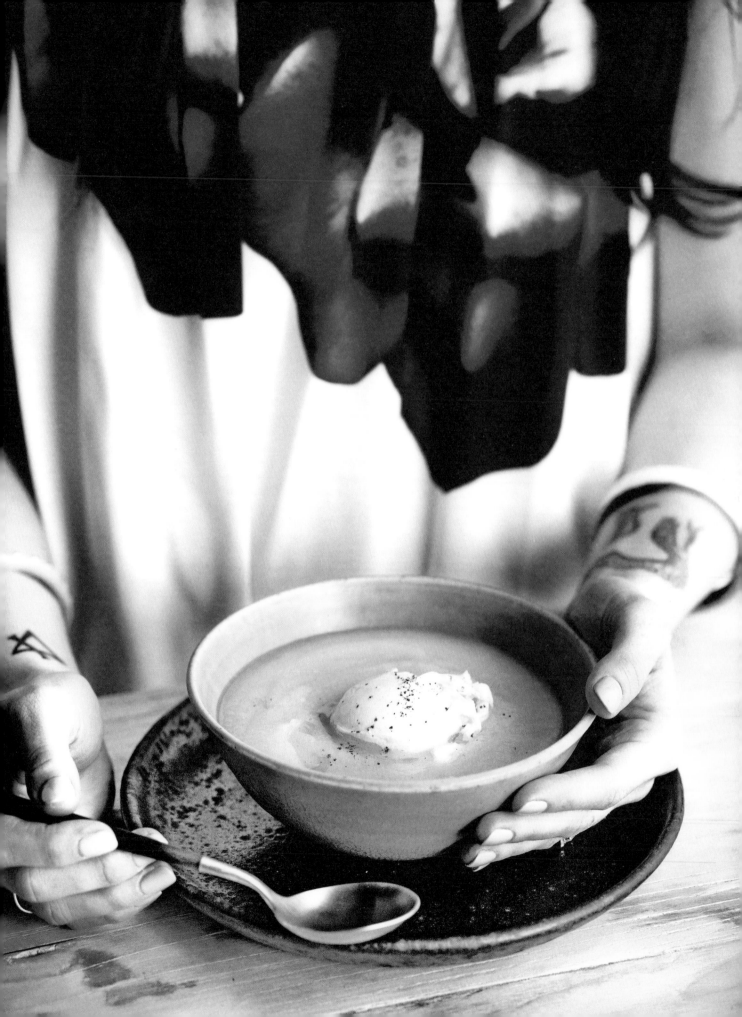

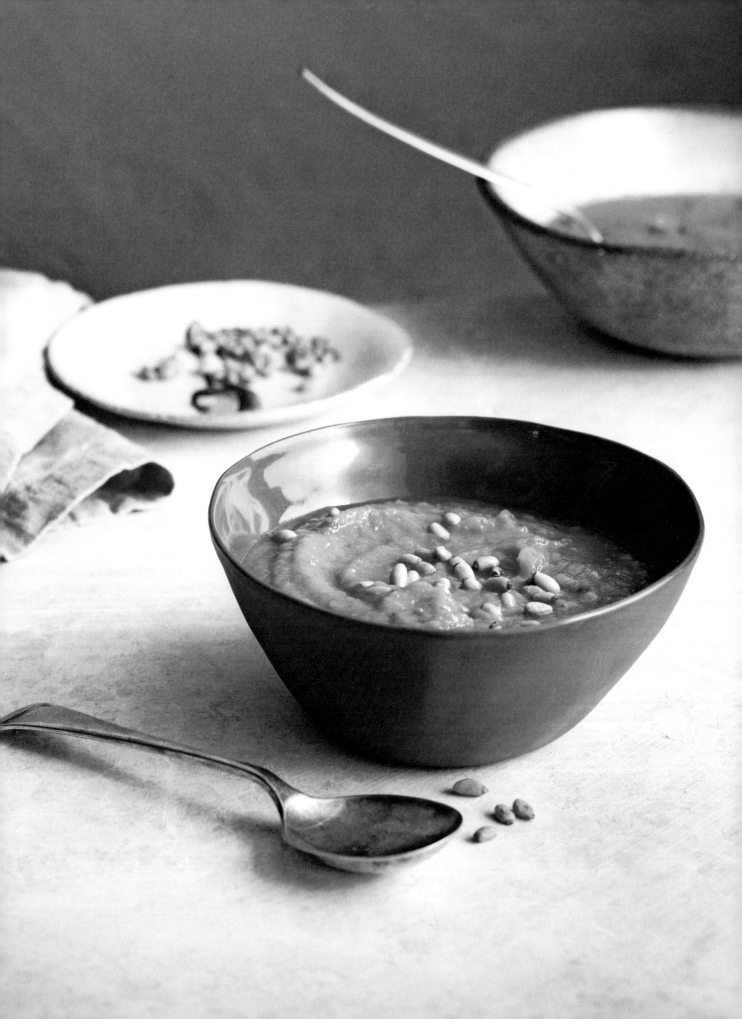

ROAST PUMPKIN, CUMIN *and* CHILLI SOUP *with* PINE NUTS

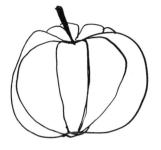

TOBIE At home, we call this soup 'I can't believe it's not butter!', because that's what a friend of mine said when I served it to him. It's absolutely delicious and with under a tablespoon of olive oil per serve, it's a winner on the health front, too. You can use any pumpkin variety, but I think that kent (jap) pumpkin works best. Back in the day I would have served it with a cheesy crouton, which would have brought the texture a pureed soup often needs. But with croutons banished, I find that nuts, or a seed and nut mix, bring all the texture and flavour one could ask for.

GEORGIA When it's cold and wintry outside I like nothing better than curling up with a bowl of this soup. Tobie and I spike it pretty heavily with chilli, which ups the warming factor even more, but we're huge chilli fans so don't feel you have to follow suit. If it's too hot for you, reduce the number of chillies, use a milder variety, remove the seeds or leave them out altogether.

Preheat the oven to 180°C. Line a baking tray with baking paper.

Place the pumpkin in a large bowl, drizzle with the extra virgin olive oil and season generously with salt and pepper, then toss to coat. Spread the pumpkin in a single layer over the lined tray and roast for 40 minutes or until golden and tender.

About 10 minutes before the pumpkin is ready, heat the olive oil in a large heavy-based saucepan or stockpot over high heat. Add the onion, celery and carrot and cook, stirring often, for 5 minutes. Reduce the heat to medium and add the garlic, chilli, rosemary, cumin and bay leaves and cook, stirring, for a further 5 minutes.

When the pumpkin is cooked, remove it from the oven and add to the pan. Pour 2 litres of water into the pan and bring to the boil over high heat, then reduce the heat and hold at a gentle simmer for 40 minutes or until all the vegetables are tender.

Remove the bay leaves, then use a blender, stick blender or food processor to blend the soup to a smooth puree. (If using a food processor or blender, cool the soup slightly before processing and do it in batches.) Taste and adjust the seasoning with salt and pepper as necessary. Reheat over low–medium heat. Ladle into serving bowls and serve scattered with the pine nuts or seed and nut mix.

SERVES: 8	
	PER SERVE
ENERGY (KJ/CAL)	865/207
PROTEIN (G)	4
FAT (G)	12
SATURATED FAT (G)	1.5
CARBOHYDRATE (G)	18

2 kg pumpkin (squash), peeled, seeds removed and cut into large chunks

2 tablespoons extra virgin olive oil

sea salt and cracked black pepper

2 tablespoons olive oil

2 red onions, roughly chopped

2 stalks celery, trimmed and roughly chopped

2 carrots, roughly chopped

3 cloves garlic, finely chopped

2 red bird's-eye chillies, halved

small handful of rosemary leaves, roughly chopped

1 teaspoon ground cumin

2 bay leaves

2 tablespoons toasted pine nuts or Seed and nut mix (see page 190), to serve

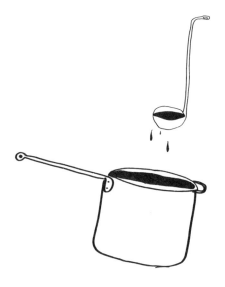

CAVOLO NERO *and* CANNELLINI BEAN SOUP

SERVES: 6

	PER SERVE
ENERGY (KJ/CAL)	906/217
PROTEIN (G)	8.5
FAT (G)	13
SATURATED FAT (G)	2.5
CARBOHYDRATE (G)	13.5

2½ tablespoons olive oil

2 stalks celery, trimmed and finely diced

2 carrots, finely diced

1 large onion, finely diced

6 cloves garlic, finely chopped

1 red bird's-eye chilli, finely chopped

3 bay leaves

200 g tinned tomatoes (preferably cherry tomatoes)

400 g tin cannellini beans, rinsed and drained

1.2 litres gluten-free vegetable stock or water

200 g trimmed cavolo nero (Tuscan kale), finely shredded

sea salt and cracked black pepper

freshly grated parmesan, to serve

extra virgin olive oil, for drizzling

TOBIE One of my favourite soups is *ribollita*, a Tuscan soup made with cavolo nero and white beans and thickened with day-old bread, which is always served with lashings of cold-pressed olive oil. For this recipe, I have taken the flavours from *ribollita*, but said goodbye to the bread and copious amounts of oil.

GEORGIA This is a very hearty, filling soup that really hits the spot in the colder months, or any time you need something comforting.

Heat the olive oil in a large heavy-based saucepan or stockpot over high heat. Add the celery, carrot, onion, garlic, chilli and bay leaves and cook, stirring often, for 10 minutes or until the vegetables start to soften.

Stir in the tomatoes and cook for 5 minutes before adding the beans and stock or water. Bring to a simmer, then reduce the heat and hold at a gentle simmer for 20 minutes.

Add the cavolo nero to the pan and cook, stirring occasionally, for 10 minutes or until the cavolo nero has softened. Remove the bay leaves.

Season with salt and pepper and serve hot with a sprinkling of parmesan and a light drizzle of extra virgin olive oil.

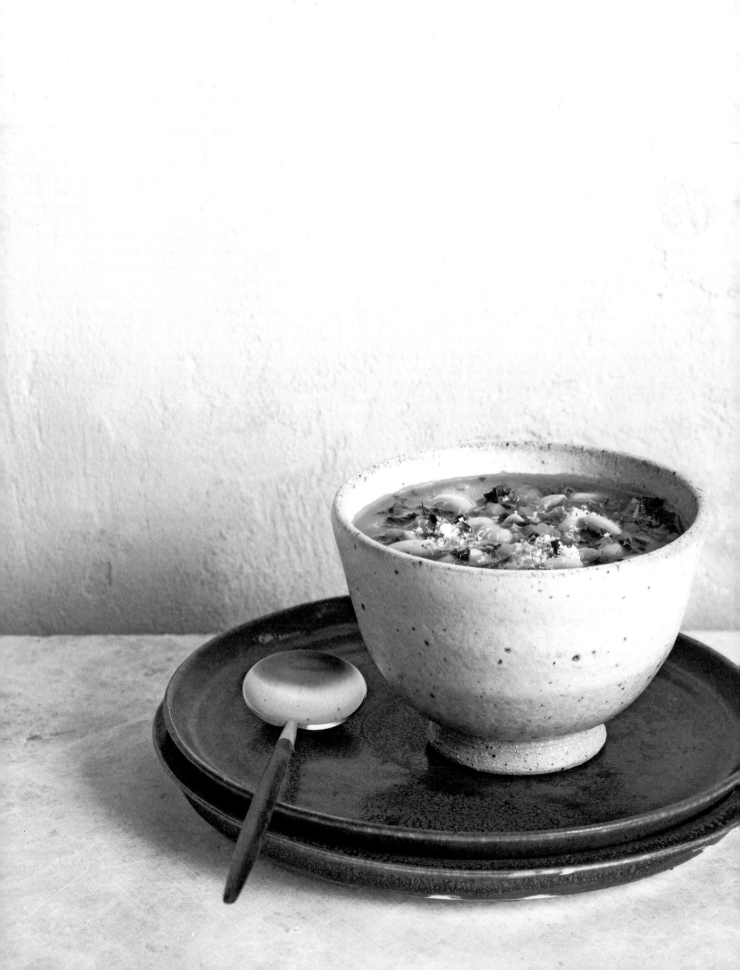

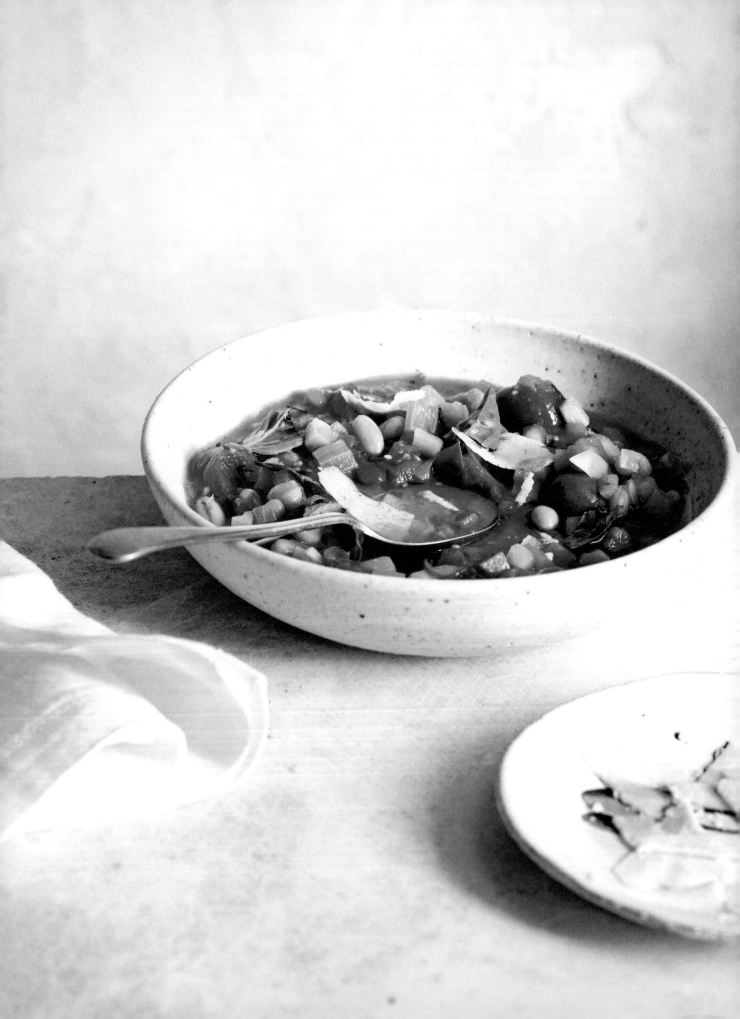

MINESTRONE

SERVES: 6

	PER SERVE
ENERGY (KJ/CAL)	1185/283
PROTEIN (G)	13
FAT (G)	13
SATURATED FAT (G)	2.5
CARBOHYDRATE (G)	23

TOBIE This soup is a 100 per cent go-to meal for Georgia and me. About once a month I make a massive batch and then freeze serving-size portions in airtight containers. It's moves like this that will save you on those nights when you don't have anything prepared or you get home late. We often serve this with a dash of truffle oil, added just before we tuck in.

Heat the olive oil in a large heavy-based saucepan or stockpot over high heat. Add the onion, carrot, celery, parsnip, rosemary, bay leaves and chilli, if using, and cook, stirring often, for 5 minutes, until the vegetables are softened slightly, but not coloured.

Add the tomatoes and cook for a further 2 minutes before adding the stock or water. Bring to the boil, then reduce the heat and hold at a gentle simmer for 30 minutes. Add the cannellini beans and simmer gently for a further 1 hour. Remove the bay leaves.

Season the soup with salt and pepper, to taste, and serve hot with a drizzle of extra virgin olive oil and a little parmesan and torn basil.

¼ cup (60 ml) extra virgin olive oil, plus extra for drizzling

1 onion, diced

1 carrot, diced

2 stalks celery, trimmed and diced

2 parsnips, peeled and diced

small handful of rosemary leaves, roughly chopped

2 bay leaves

1 red bird's-eye chilli, finely chopped (optional)

400 g tin cherry tomatoes or chopped tomatoes

1.5 litres gluten-free vegetable or chicken stock, or water

2 × 400 g tins cannellini beans, rinsed and drained

sea salt and cracked black pepper

shaved parmesan, to serve

basil leaves, to serve

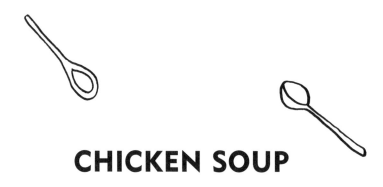

CHICKEN SOUP

SERVES: 4–6

	PER SERVE (FOR 6)
ENERGY (KJ/CAL)	1183/286
PROTEIN (G)	29
FAT (G)	15
SATURATED FAT (G)	4.5
CARBOHYDRATE (G)	6

1 × 1.4 kg chicken

1 onion, thinly sliced

1 carrot, diagonally sliced

2 stalks celery, trimmed and diagonally sliced

1 leek, white part only, washed well and thinly sliced

3 cloves garlic, thinly sliced

3 bay leaves

2 sprigs sage

1 teaspoon black peppercorns

2 cups (320 g) fresh or frozen peas

sea salt

freshly grated parmesan, to serve

TOBIE This is a beautifully simple dish, in terms of both preparation and flavour. Get the best-quality chicken you can afford. I use water in this recipe and it becomes a stock during the cooking process, but you could use stock initially to intensify the chicken flavour. If you have some muslin, wrap the bay leaves, sage and peppercorns in it – this makes them easier to remove at the end.

GEORGIA I've been pescetarian (fish-eating vegetarian) for the last 10 years, but I must admit I tasted this soup as it brought back memories of my nana Freda's chicken soup, which was sublime.

Place the chicken in a large heavy-based saucepan or stockpot with the onion, carrot, celery, leek, garlic, bay leaves, sage and peppercorns. Add enough cold water to submerge the chicken (about 3 litres). Bring to the boil over high heat, then reduce the heat and hold at a gentle simmer.

After 1½ hours the chicken will be cooked and you will have a wonderful chicken stock. Turn off the heat, then very carefully transfer the chicken to a plate or large bowl and set aside until it's cool enough to handle. Use your fingers to shred the chicken meat, discarding the skin and bones.

Skim the fat from the surface of the stock if necessary, then bring to a gentle simmer. Add the peas and shredded chicken to the pan and simmer for a further minute before removing from the heat. Taste and season with salt. Use a slotted spoon to remove the bay leaves, sage and peppercorns. Serve the soup topped with a good pinch of parmesan.

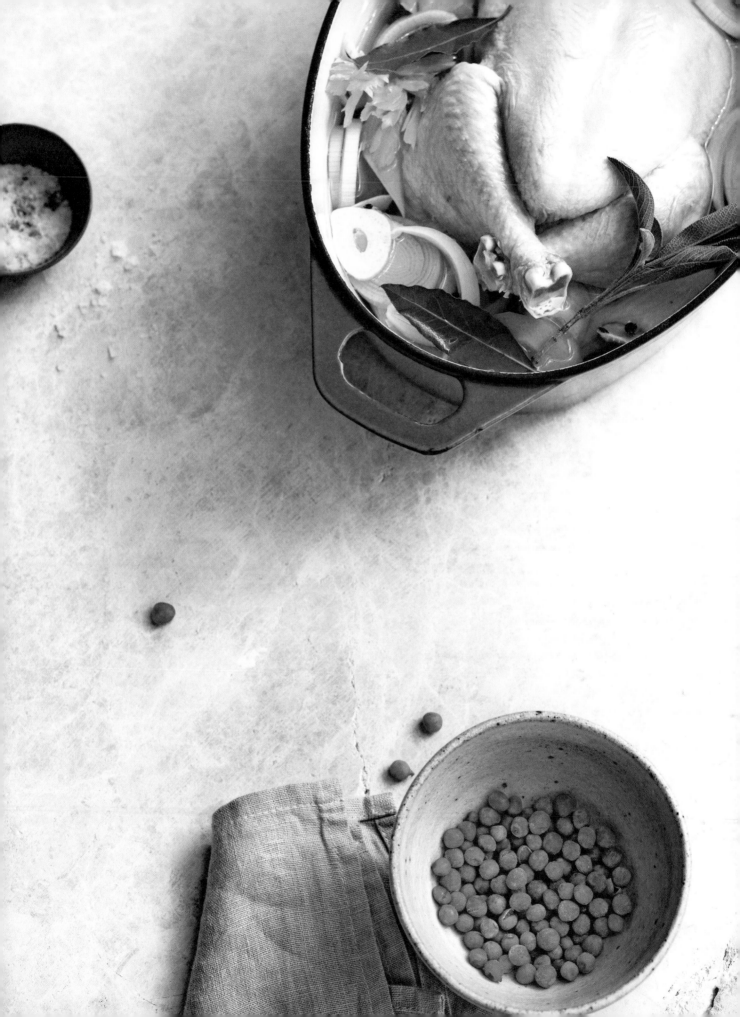

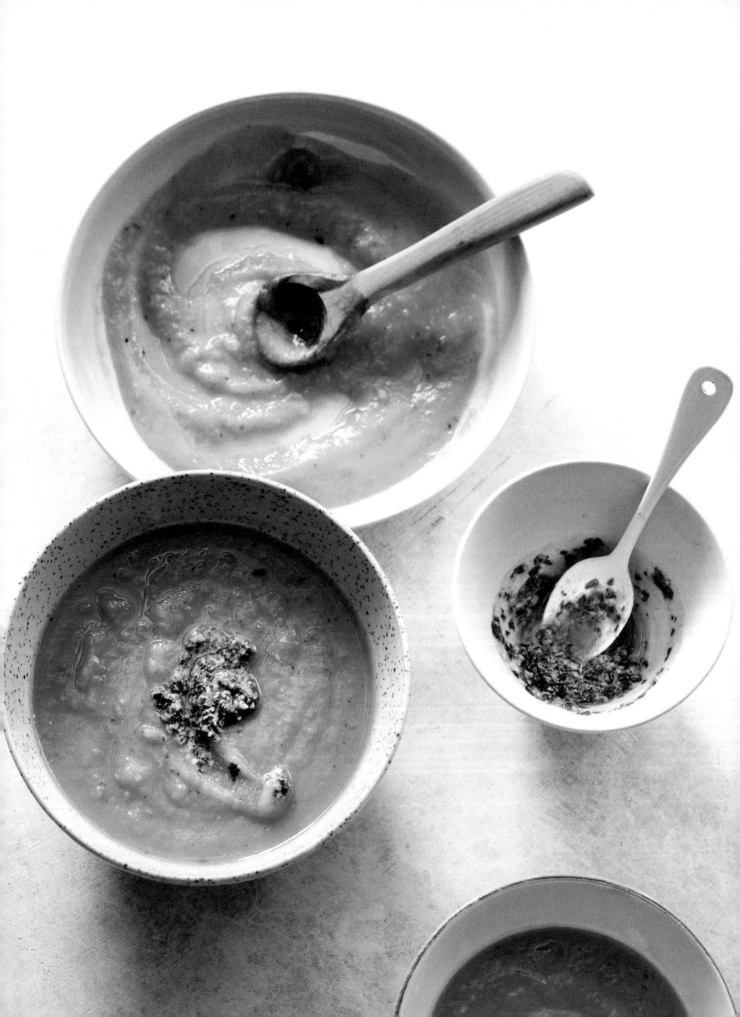

ROASTED SWEET POTATO and GARLIC SOUP with BASIL PESTO

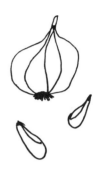

TOBIE There's a truckload of flavour in this soup, with the caramelised sweetness of the roasted sweet potato and the nutty, herby hit from the pesto. You could use a commercial pesto instead of making your own if you're short of time – just check the label to make sure it's gluten free. (If you make your own pesto you don't have to worry, as it's gluten-free by nature.)

Preheat the oven to 200°C. Line a large baking tray with baking paper.

Place the sweet potato in a bowl and add a good pinch of both salt and pepper. Drizzle in 1 tablespoon of the olive oil and add the unpeeled garlic cloves. Toss to combine, then spread out over the lined tray. Bake for 30–40 minutes or until the sweet potato is tender and starting to darken in colour. Remove from the oven and carefully peel the garlic cloves.

Meanwhile, heat the remaining olive oil in a large, heavy-based saucepan or stockpot over low–medium heat. Add the onion, carrot, celery and thyme and cook, stirring often, for 10 minutes or until softened.

Increase the heat to medium, add the garlic and sweet potato and cook, stirring often, for 2 minutes. Add the stock or water and bring to the boil over high heat, then reduce the heat and hold at a simmer for 30 minutes. Puree the soup using a blender, stick blender or food processor, then season with salt and pepper, to taste. (If using a food processor or blender, cool the soup slightly before processing and do it in batches.)

Serve topped with a teaspoon of basil pesto.

SERVES: 4–6

	PER SERVE (FOR 6)
ENERGY (KJ/CAL)	1330/318
PROTEIN (G)	8
FAT (G)	14
SATURATED FAT (G)	2
CARBOHYDRATE (G)	38

1.2 kg sweet potato, peeled and cut into 2 cm cubes

sea salt and cracked black pepper

¼ cup (60 ml) extra virgin olive oil

6 cloves garlic, unpeeled

1 onion, roughly chopped

1 carrot, roughly chopped

2 stalks celery, trimmed and roughly chopped

1 heaped tablespoon thyme leaves

2.5 litres gluten-free vegetable stock or water

Basil pesto (see page 185), to serve

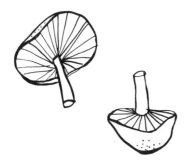

MUSHROOM *and* LEEK SOUP

SERVES: 4

	PER SERVE
ENERGY (KJ/CAL)	703/168
PROTEIN (G)	8
FAT (G)	11.5
SATURATED FAT (G)	2.5
CARBOHYDRATE (G)	6.5

2 tablespoons extra virgin olive oil

1 onion, finely diced

1 stalk celery, trimmed and finely diced

1 large leek, white part only, washed well and thinly sliced

4 cloves garlic, thinly sliced

small handful of rosemary leaves, roughly chopped

2 bay leaves

500 g mushrooms, wiped clean with paper towel and sliced

1 litre gluten-free stock (vegetable or chicken) or water

shaved parmesan, to serve

extra virgin olive oil, chilli oil or truffle oil, to serve (optional)

TOBIE Unlike traditional mushroom soup, there is no cream or butter in this version. I like to use a combination of mushrooms, like button, field and swiss, or whatever's around at the time, but you could really use whatever you want. As for the stock, chicken stock is fantastic in this dish, however vegetable stock also works well and much of the time I even use council stock (water!).

Heat the olive oil in a large heavy-based saucepan or stockpot over medium heat. Add the onion, celery, leek, garlic, rosemary and bay leaves and cook, stirring often, for about 10 minutes or until the onion is soft and translucent, without any colouring. You may need to reduce the heat to low – what's important here is the texture of the onion, not the timing.

Once the vegetables are soft, increase the heat to high and add the mushrooms. Cook, stirring, for 5 minutes or until the mushrooms begin to brown. Add the stock or water and bring to the boil, then reduce the heat and hold at a simmer for 30 minutes. Remove the bay leaves.

Use a blender, stick blender or food processor to briefly process the soup – you want to retain some texture so don't turn it into a puree. (If using a food processor or blender, cool the soup slightly before processing and do it in batches.)

Serve with a cheeky sprinkling of parmesan and a drizzle of olive, chilli or truffle oil.

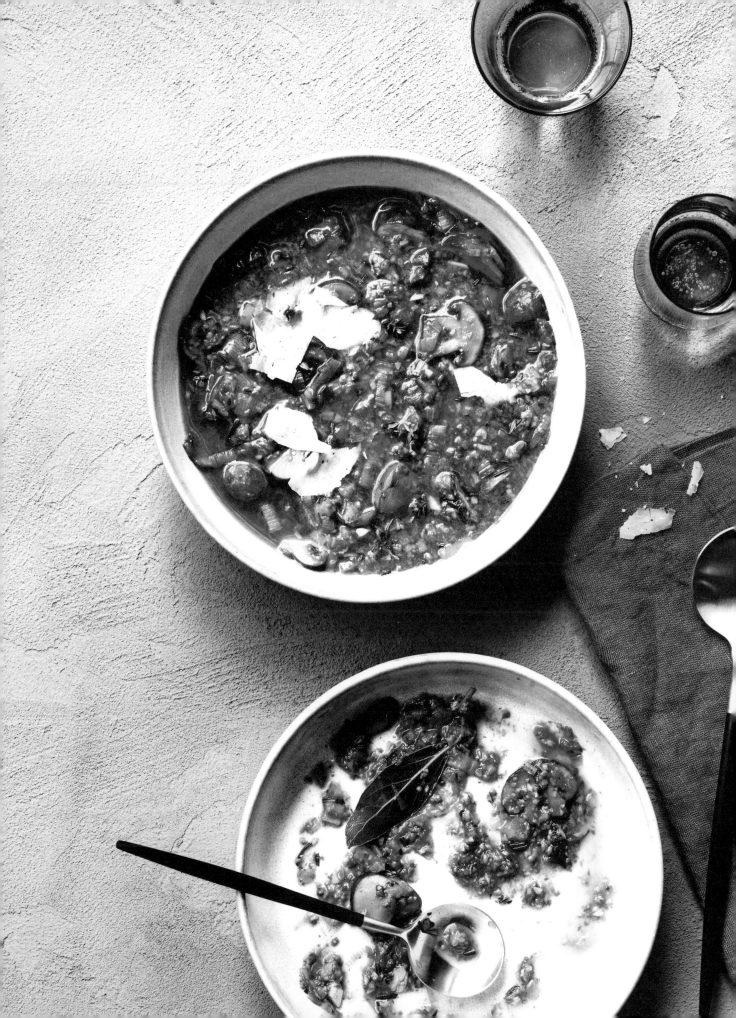

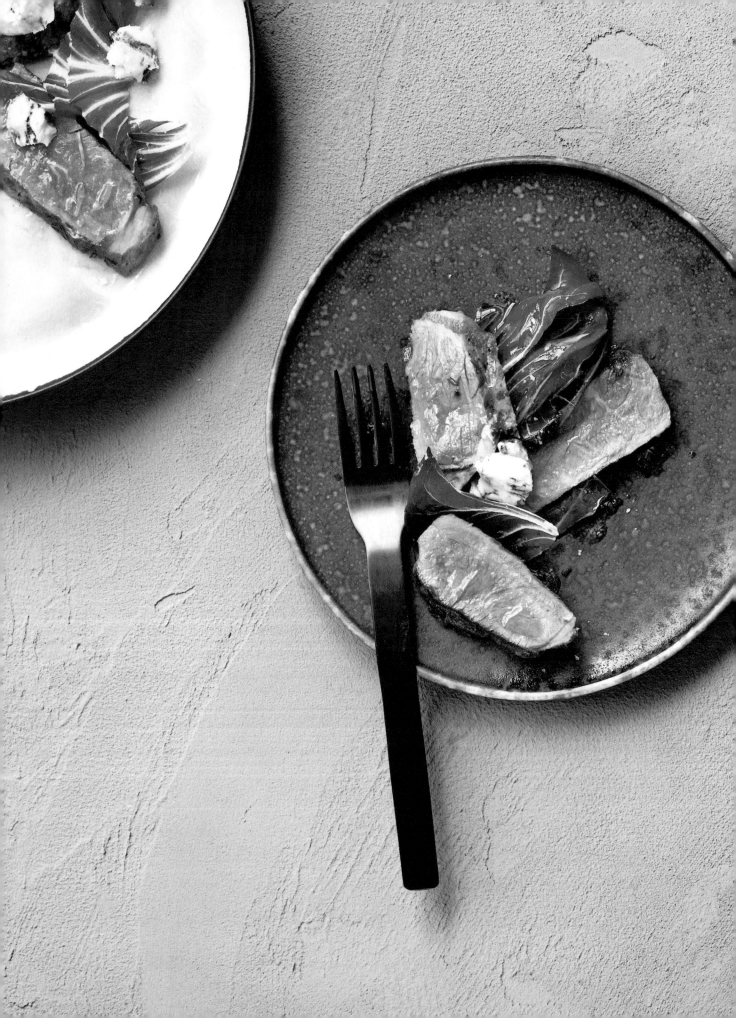

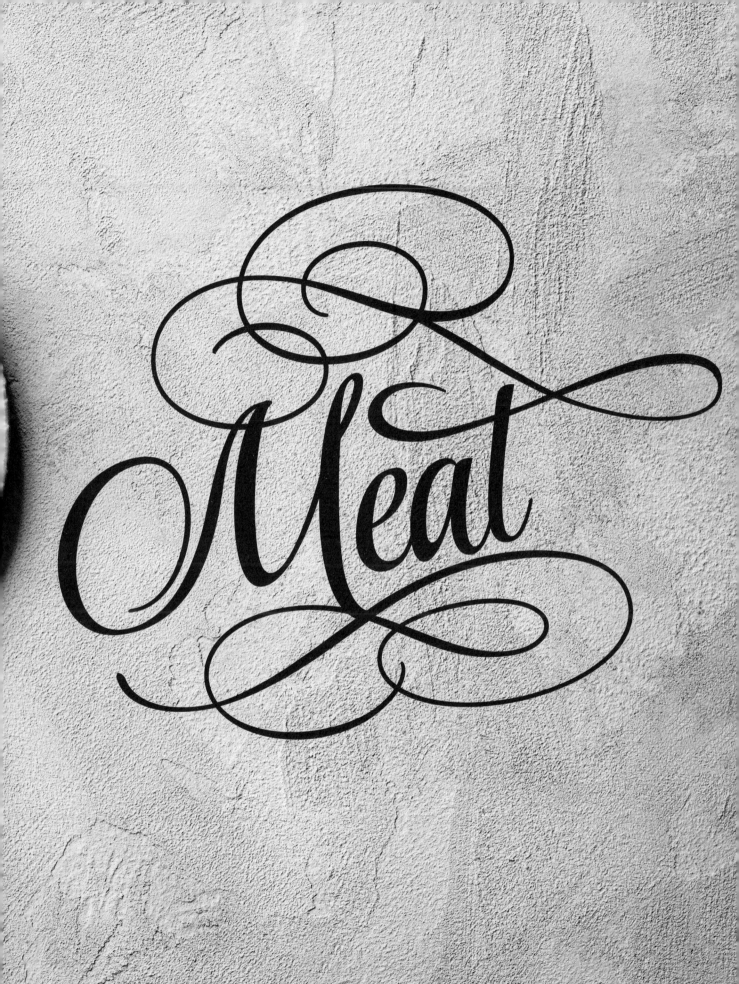

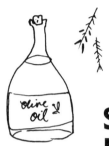

SLOW-ROASTED LAMB SHOULDER

SERVES: 4-6

	PER SERVE (FOR 6)
ENERGY (KJ/CAL)	1434/343
PROTEIN (G)	41.5
FAT (G)	18
SATURATED FAT (G)	7.5
CARBOHYDRATE (G)	2.5

olive oil, to grease

1 tablespoon fennel seeds

4 sprigs rosemary, leaves picked

4 cloves garlic, peeled

sea salt and cracked black pepper

12 anchovy fillets

2 tablespoons extra virgin olive oil

1.5 kg lamb shoulder on the bone, fat trimmed

2 red onions, thickly sliced

TOBIE This is a dish that could easily turn the corner and not be suitable for this book because of all the gorgeous fat that gathers in the bottom of the pan. I used to roast potatoes in it or make a sauce – you name it, I'd do it! But I won't be using it here so that you can enjoy the superb flavour of a lamb roast without sabotaging your healthy eating habits.

Preheat the oven to the highest temperature possible. Lightly grease a roasting pan with olive oil.

Toast the fennel seeds in a dry frying pan over medium heat for a couple of minutes, until aromatic. Transfer to a mortar and add the rosemary leaves, garlic and a good pinch of salt. Use the pestle to pound to a paste and then work in the anchovies. Add the extra virgin olive oil to bring the mixture to a loose paste consistency.

Use a sharp knife to make some long, diagonal incisions into the fat side of the lamb and then rub the anchovy mixture into the incisions. Scatter the sliced onion over the base of the roasting pan, lay the lamb on top and then cover tightly with foil.

Place in the oven and turn the heat down to 160°C. Roast for 5 hours, by which time the meat should be falling apart really easily. If it's not, just cook it for a little longer. If the base of the pan gets a bit dry during the long cooking time, just add a little water.

Remove the lamb from the oven and leave to rest for about 10 minutes before transferring to a large chopping board. Use a couple of forks to pull the meat off the bone and shred it as you go. Serve with the onion.

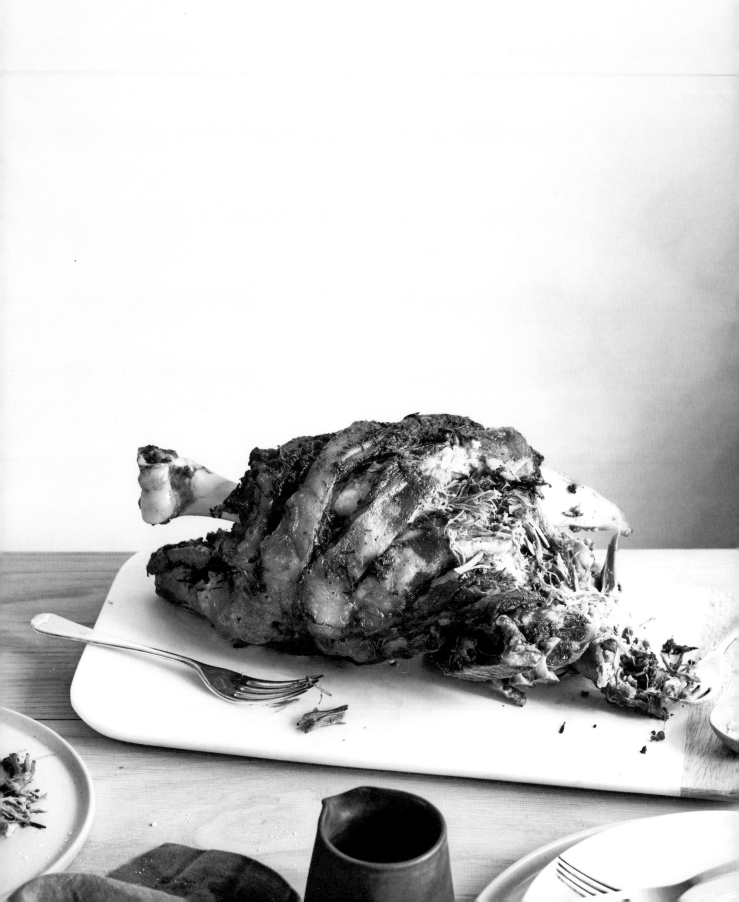

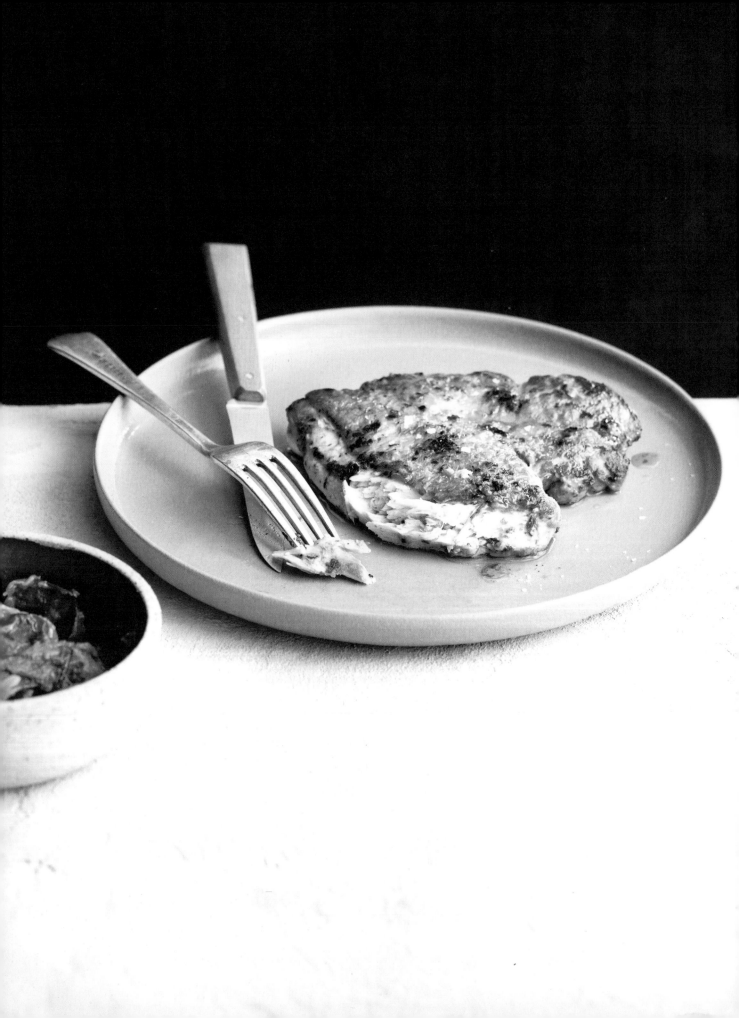

CHICKEN *with* MARJORAM, FENNEL SEEDS *and* CHILLI

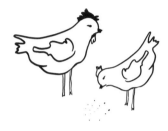

SERVES: 4

	PER SERVE
ENERGY (KJ/CAL)	1699/406
PROTEIN (G)	51.5
FAT (G)	21.5
SATURATED FAT (G)	5.5
CARBOHYDRATE (G)	0.5

TOBIE I also like to cook this dish in the Italian style of *al mattone*, meaning 'under a brick'. To do this, when you put the chicken on the grill you place a piece of baking paper on top of it and then a brick large enough to cover the entire chicken goes on top of that. This flattens the chicken, which encourages it to cook a little quicker and as a result the chicken retains much of the moisture that is otherwise lost with longer cooking times.

Place the boned chicken or fillets on a chopping board, cover with plastic film and gently bash with a meat mallet or rolling pin until around 1 cm thick.

Put the garlic, marjoram, lemon zest, fennel seeds, chilli and a pinch of salt into a mortar and pound with the pestle to a coarse paste. Add the olive oil to loosen the mixture and season with pepper.

Put the chicken in a glass or ceramic dish and use your hands to rub the marinade all over both sides. Cover and place in the fridge to marinate for up to 12 hours (the longer the better, but if you are in a rush you can also cook it right away). Remove from the fridge 30 minutes before cooking.

Preheat a barbecue, grill plate or chargrill pan on high. When it is very hot, place the chicken on it and cook for 8–10 minutes each side, until the juices run clear when a skewer is inserted into the thickest part. While the chicken is cooking, cut the zested lemon in half and place, flesh side down, on the barbecue or grill.

Serve the chicken right away with the grilled lemon and a drizzle of extra virgin olive oil, if desired.

1 × 1.4 kg butterflied and boned chicken, halved or 4 chicken breast fillets, skin on

2 small cloves garlic, peeled

small handful of marjoram leaves

finely grated zest of 1 lemon

1 teaspoon fennel seeds

1 red bird's-eye chilli, finely chopped

sea salt and cracked black pepper

1 tablespoon extra virgin olive oil, plus extra for drizzling (optional)

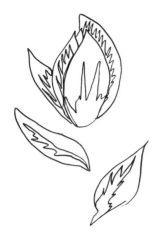

TAGLIATA DI MANZO with GORGONZOLA and RADICCHIO

SERVES: 4

	PER SERVE
ENERGY (KJ/CAL)	2036/487
PROTEIN (G)	51.5
FAT (G)	30
SATURATED FAT (G)	10.5
CARBOHYDRATE (G)	2

4 × 200 g beef sirloin steaks

¼ cup (60 ml) extra virgin olive oil

2 sprigs rosemary, leaves picked

sea salt and cracked black pepper

3 lemons, halved

1 large head of radicchio, washed and roughly chopped (or 4 handfuls of rocket)

80 g gorgonzola or soft goat's cheese

TOBIE *Tagliata di manzo* means 'cut beef' and it's commonly served with rocket leaves, lemon and extra virgin olive oil. It's essentially Italian steak and salad. This version calls on a couple of different flavours. The radicchio is slightly bitter, while the gorgonzola is a little sweet, and these two, married with a good extra virgin olive oil, take me straight to my happy place. Gorgonzola is a rather fatty cheese, so I've allocated just 20 g per person, however the strong flavour goes a long way. It could be replaced with cottage cheese or a low-fat ricotta if you prefer. Remember that simple dishes with just a few ingredients, like this, rely 100 per cent on the quality of the produce.

Put the beef, 1 tablespoon olive oil, the rosemary and a pinch of pepper in a glass or ceramic dish, mix well and set aside for 20–30 minutes to marinate.

Preheated the barbecue or grill plate on high.

Remove the beef from the marinade and shake it a little to remove any excess oil. When the barbecue or grill is super-hot, place the beef on it along with 4 of the lemon halves, flesh side down. Cook the beef for 1–2 minutes on each side or until cooked to your liking, then transfer to a plate and set aside for a minute or so to rest. By this time the lemons should be nice and caramelised, so transfer them to a separate plate also.

Meanwhile, pop the radicchio into a bowl and dress with 1 tablespoon of olive oil and a squeeze of lemon juice from the uncooked lemon halves.

Slice the steaks as thinly as you like – I like mine to be around 5 mm thick. Pop the sliced meat and any juices into a bowl, add the remaining tablespoon of olive oil and a pinch of salt, and toss the meat so the olive oil and salt are distributed evenly.

Arrange the meat on serving plates or one large platter and distribute the radicchio around and under it. Break the gorgonzola or goat's cheese into little chunks and scatter over the meat. Serve immediately with the grilled lemon halves.

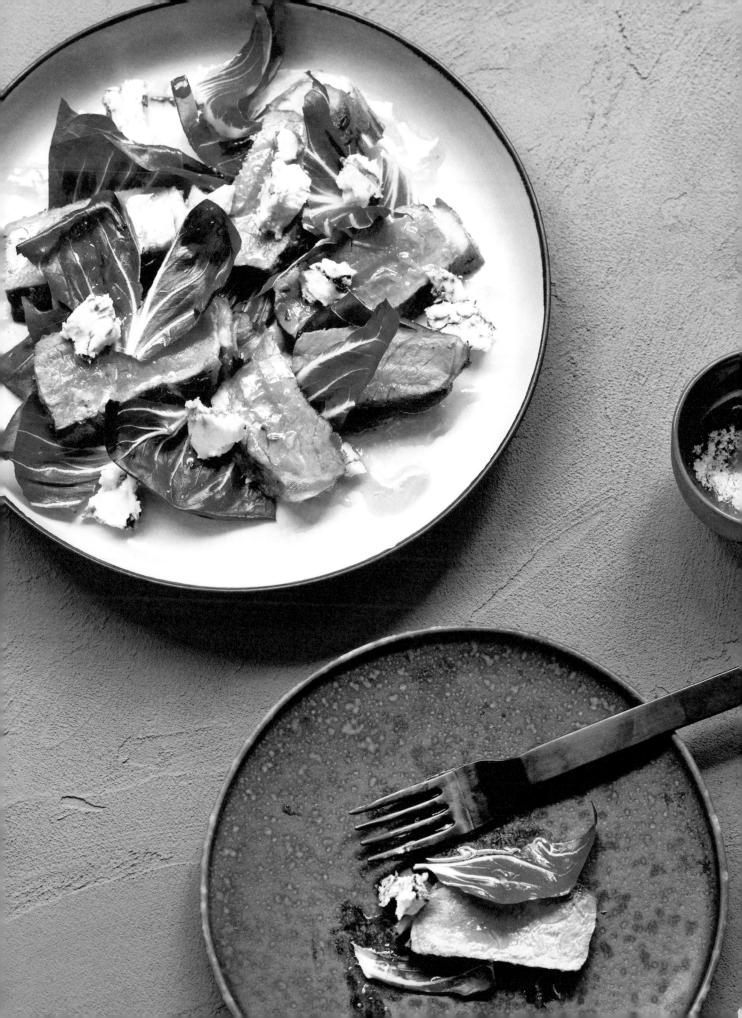

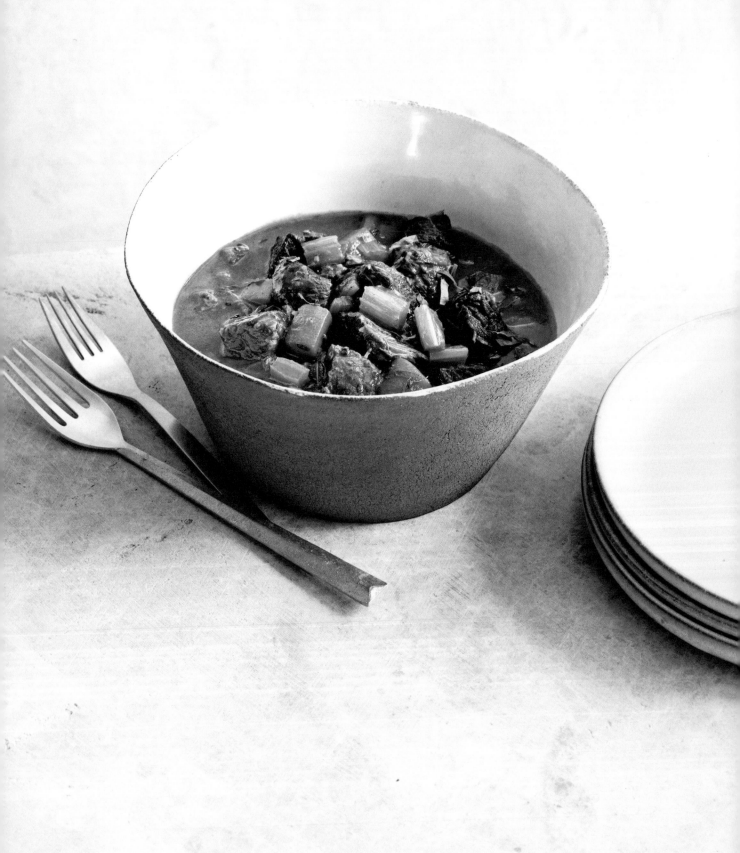

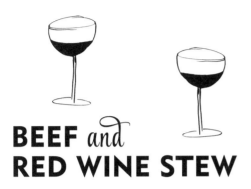

BEEF and RED WINE STEW

SERVES: 4

	PER SERVE
ENERGY (KJ/CAL)	2231/534
PROTEIN (G)	54
FAT (G)	26
SATURATED FAT (G)	6.5
CARBOHYDRATE (G)	12

TOBIE This rich, luxurious, comforting stew is surprisingly light on the hips and the orange zest really lifts it to another level.

Heat half the olive oil in a large flameproof casserole dish over high heat. Dust the beef with the flour and cook in 2–3 batches, until sealed. Transfer the beef to a bowl as each batch is sealed and set aside.

Heat the remaining olive oil in the casserole dish over low–medium heat and gently cook the onion, celery, carrot, garlic, rosemary, chilli, if using, bay leaves and sage for about 15 minutes, until the vegetables are softened. Stir every couple of minutes to prevent anything sticking to the base of the dish.

Return the meat to the dish and cook over high heat for a couple of minutes, until browned. Add the wine and cook until it has almost reduced completely, then add the stock or water, and tomatoes. Stir to mix well.

Cover the dish, reduce the heat to low and simmer gently for 2–3 hours. To test whether the stew is ready, pull a little piece of beef out and press on it lightly with a fork – if it falls apart, it is tender and ready to go. It's important that there is ample moisture in the dish during the cooking process, so if it looks like it's becoming dry, add more stock or water.

Taste the stew and season with salt and pepper, then stir in the parsley and orange zest and finish with a drizzle of extra virgin olive oil, if you like.

¼ cup (60 ml) extra virgin olive oil, plus extra for drizzling (optional)

1 kg beef shoulder (chuck), cut into 3 cm cubes

gluten-free plain flour, for dusting

2 onions, roughly chopped

3 stalks celery, trimmed and roughly chopped

3 carrots, roughly chopped

2 cloves garlic, finely chopped

handful of rosemary leaves, roughly chopped

1 red bird's-eye chilli, chopped (optional)

2 bay leaves

10 sage leaves

1 cup (250 ml) red wine

2 cups (500 ml) gluten-free beef stock or water, approximately

400 g tin chopped tomatoes

sea salt and cracked black pepper

large handful of flat-leaf parsley, roughly chopped

finely grated zest of 1 orange

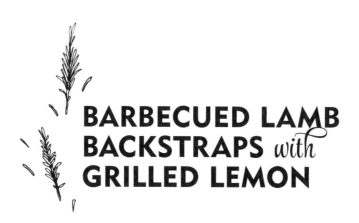

BARBECUED LAMB BACKSTRAPS *with* GRILLED LEMON

SERVES: 4

	PER SERVE
ENERGY (KJ/CAL)	1353/324
PROTEIN (G)	43.5
FAT (G)	16
SATURATED FAT (G)	4.5
CARBOHYDRATE (G)	0.5

2 × 400 g lamb backstraps, trimmed of any sinew

2 cloves garlic, finely chopped

small handful of rosemary leaves

finely grated zest and juice of 1 lemon

1 tablespoon olive oil

sea salt and cracked black pepper

2 lemons, halved

TOBIE This cut of lamb is often overlooked, but I really love it. You can marinate it in all sorts of flavours or cook it sous vide, but the purpose of this book is to bring you simple, healthy and delicious recipes, so here is a straightforward lemon, garlic, rosemary and lamb dish. Here, we've served it with the Kale with chilli, garlic and lemon (page 102), but it would go well with just about any of the vegetable or salad recipes in this book.

Pop the lamb in a large glass or ceramic bowl with the garlic, rosemary leaves, lemon zest and juice, and olive oil. Season with a pinch of both salt and pepper and mix until the lamb is well coated. Cover and place in the fridge for at least 1 hour to marinate (or up to 2 hours). Remove from the fridge 30 minutes before cooking.

Preheat a barbecue or grill plate on medium–high. Place the lemon halves on it, flesh side down, and cook until the flesh is quite dark in colour, about 5 minutes. Transfer to a plate and set aside.

Make sure the barbecue or grill is super-hot, then remove the lamb from the marinade, add to the barbecue or grill and cook for 3 minutes each side for medium–rare or until cooked to your liking. Transfer to a plate and set aside for 5 minutes to rest.

Thinly slice the lamb, season with pepper and serve with the grilled lemon.

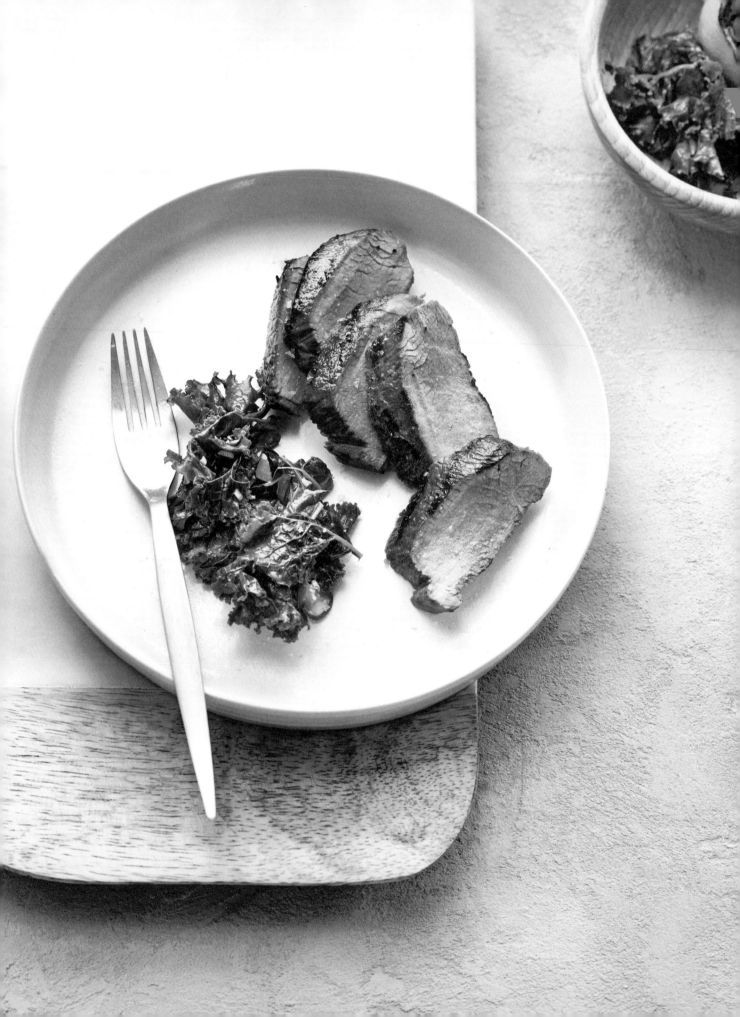

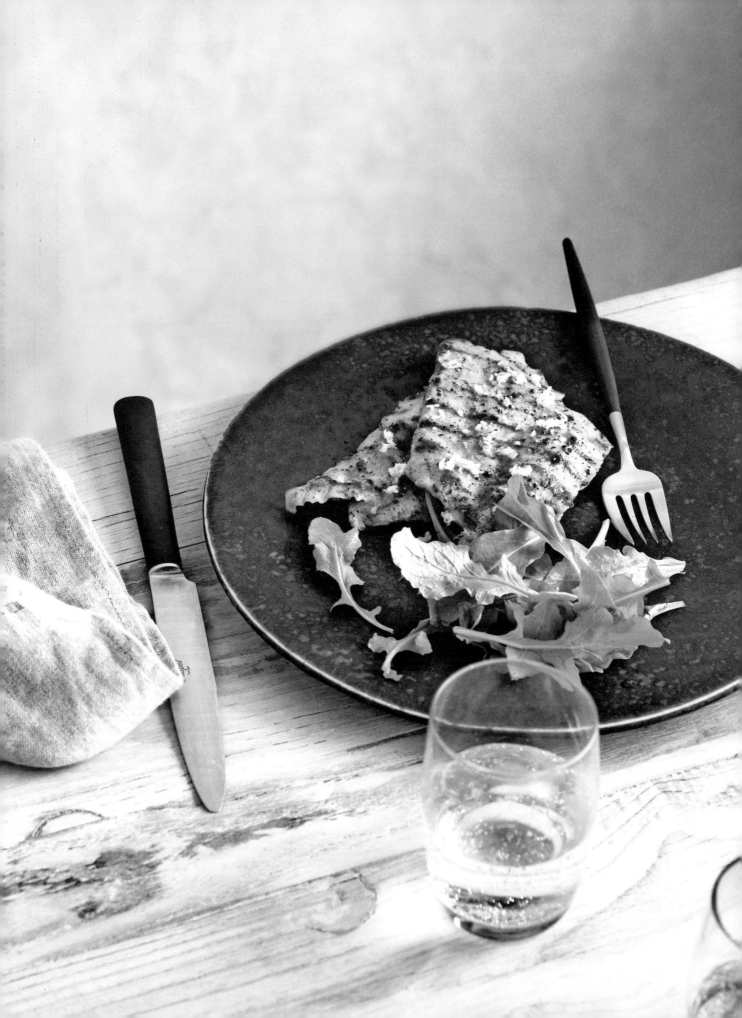

VEAL PAILLARD *with* ROCKET *and* HORSERADISH

TOBIE Considering how delicious it is, paillard (also known as escalope) often slips under the radar. Basically, it's meat (mostly chicken or veal) that is beaten until it is very thin. This tenderises it and allows it to cook very quickly – genius! The cut we're after here is the same that's used for the famous veal schnitzel, or scaloppini. Remember that you want the meat to be very thin so if it looks a bit thick, just ask your butcher to beat it until it's a little thinner or do it yourself with a meat mallet.

Preheat a barbecue, grill plate or chargrill pan on high. Put 1 tablespoon of the olive oil in a bowl, add a good pinch of salt and give it a little stir to combine. Use a pastry brush or spoon to rub the seasoned oil over the veal, making sure you coat the entire surface on both sides.

When the grill is very hot, put the lemon halves on it, flesh side down.

Meanwhile, dress the rocket in a large bowl with the remaining olive oil and a pinch of both salt and pepper. Use your hands to toss the rocket, being careful not to bruise it.

When the lemons are quite dark in colour underneath, transfer them to a plate. Add the veal to the barbecue or grill and cook for 30 seconds on each side, then transfer to a plate and leave to rest for 1 minute. Cut each piece of veal in half crossways.

Place the cooked veal on serving plates and sprinkle with pepper and horseradish. Serve immediately with rocket and grilled lemon.

SERVES: 4

	PER SERVE
ENERGY (KJ/CAL)	1259/301
PROTEIN (G)	26
FAT (G)	19
SATURATED FAT (G)	7
CARBOHYDRATE (G)	3.5

2 tablespoons extra virgin olive oil

sea salt and cracked black pepper

4 veal schnitzels or scaloppine (about 180 g each), beaten to 5 mm thick

2 lemons, halved

4 big handfuls of rocket, washed and dried

1 tablespoon freshly grated horseradish

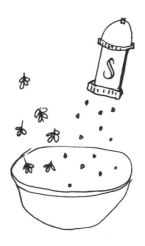

ROAST CHICKEN
with SAGE *and* LEMON

SERVES: 4

	PER SERVE
ENERGY (KJ/CAL)	1834/439
PROTEIN (G)	53
FAT (G)	19
SATURATED FAT (G)	5
CARBOHYDRATE (G)	4.5

10 sage leaves

1 lemon, zest finely grated, then halved

1 tablespoon sea salt

1 × 1.4 kg chicken

1 apple, quartered and cored

4 cloves garlic, squashed

olive oil, for drizzling

2 onions, sliced

2 carrots, thickly sliced

2 stalks celery, trimmed and thickly sliced

1 cup (250 ml) white wine

TOBIE There's no molecular gastronomy here, just good humble flavours. As always, it's worth using the best-quality chicken you can afford. Slashing the legs of the chicken is a great trick that helps the marinade infuse into the meat. I often serve this with the Quinoa, broccolini and asparagus salad on page 141.

Preheat the oven to 180°C.

Put the sage, lemon zest and salt into a mortar and use the pestle to pound until you have a vibrant green salt. If it becomes too paste-like, add a little more salt until it is grainy again.

Stuff the cavity of the chicken with the apple, lemon halves and garlic, then use kitchen string to tie the drumsticks together. (This helps the bird hold its shape during cooking and also prevents the ingredients in the cavity falling out.) Slash the drumsticks a few times – this will help the flavoured salt penetrate the meat.

Drizzle a roasting pan with a little olive oil and scatter the onion, carrot and celery over the base. Place the chicken on top of the vegetables, then rub the flavoured salt over the entire surface of the chicken. Roast the chicken and vegetables for 10 minutes, then splash in the wine and cook for about 1 hour more, basting from time to time to keep the meat moist. The chicken is ready if the juices run clear when you tip it on an angle. If the juices are still pink, it is not cooked through and needs a little more time in the oven.

Remove from the oven and serve the chicken and roasted vegetables immediately, with any cooking juices spooned over.

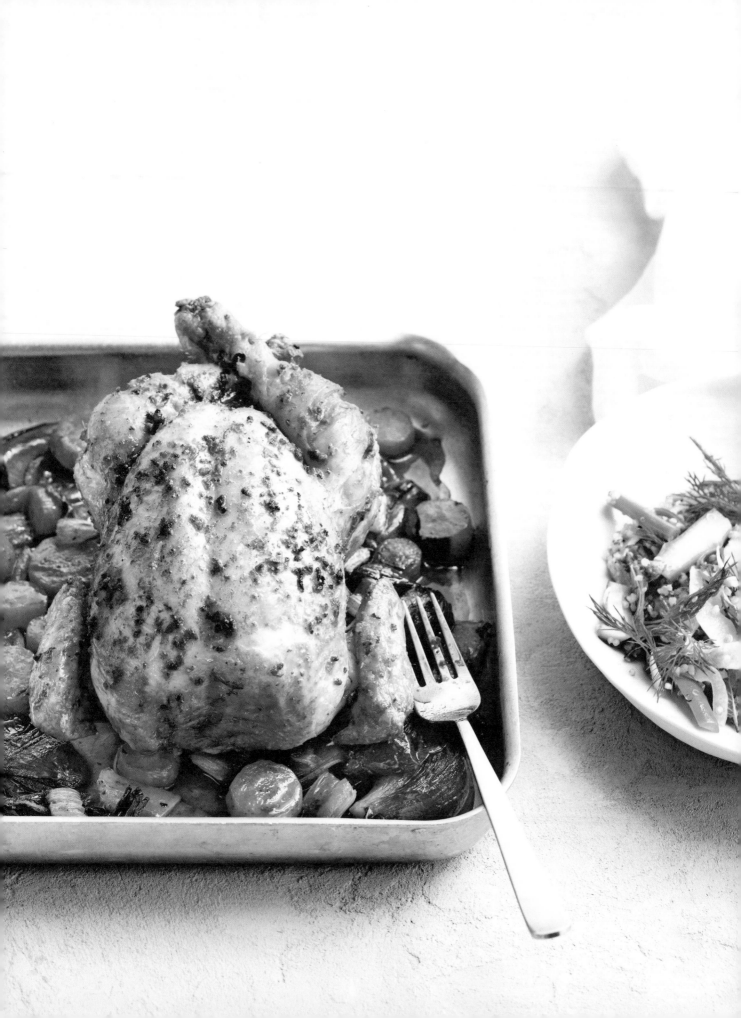

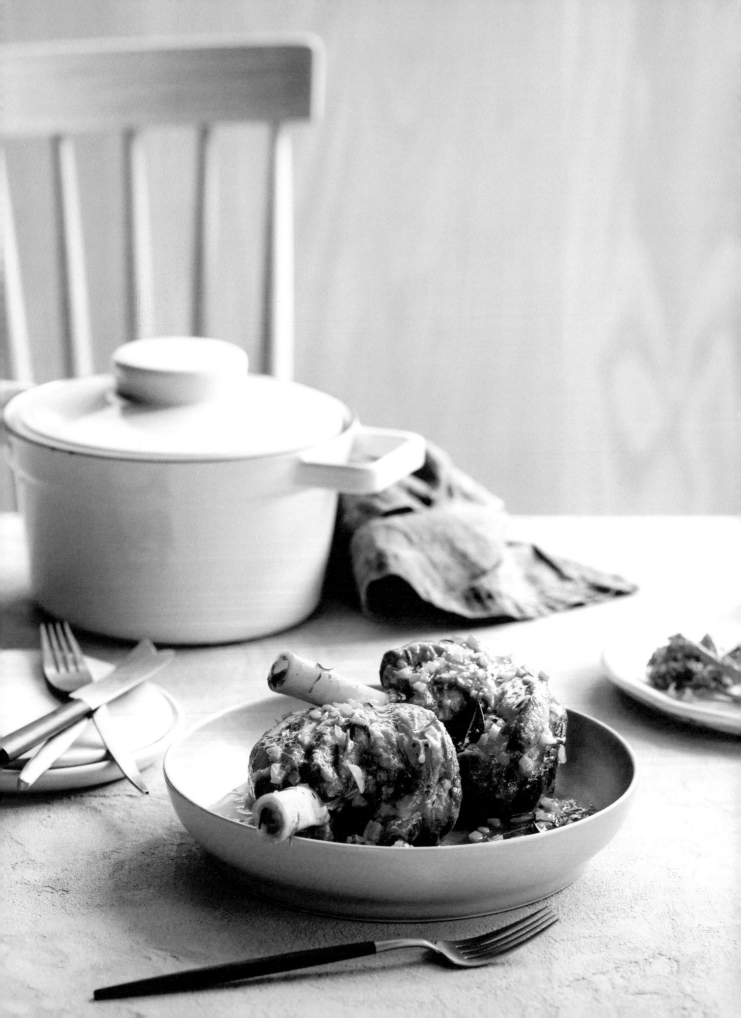

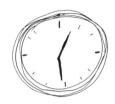

BRAISED LAMB SHANKS

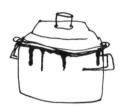

TOBIE When we changed our diet around I immediately thought of all the things I couldn't eat, like croquettes and pasta and so on. What I didn't focus on right away was the full-flavoured dishes I'd been cooking for years, like these shanks. They are braised, there's little oil and, served with a light salad or veggie dish, you have yourself a dish with a deepened flavour that still falls in the healthy camp.

SERVES: 4

	PER SERVE
ENERGY (KJ/CAL)	1389/332
PROTEIN (G)	28.5
FAT (G)	19
SATURATED FAT (G)	5
CARBOHYDRATE (G)	6

Scatter the flour over a plate, season with a good pinch of both salt and pepper and mix to combine. Dust the lamb shanks in the seasoned flour.

Heat the olive oil in a large ovenproof saucepan or flameproof casserole dish over medium–high heat. Drop a pinch of flour into the oil – if it starts sizzling, the oil is hot and ready for action. Carefully place the shanks in the pan or dish and cook for about 10 minutes, until browned all over. Remove the shanks and set aside on a plate.

Preheat the oven to 180°C.

Add the onion, carrot, celery, garlic, rosemary and bay leaves to the saucepan or dish. Reduce the heat to low and cook gently for 10 minutes or until the vegetables are soft and just starting to colour.

Increase the heat to high, add the tomato paste and cook, stirring, for 1 minute. Add the wine and cook until it has almost completely reduced, stirring to dislodge any cooked-on bits from the base of the pan or dish. Add the stock and bring to the boil, then reduce the heat and hold at a simmer.

Return the shanks to the pan or dish, cover with the lid or wrap tightly with foil, and cook in the oven for 2 hours. The lamb is ready when it comes away from the bone easily and is tender to the touch (if it's not, give it a bit more time in the oven). Remove the shanks from the pan or dish using a slotted spoon and transfer to a plate to rest.

Put the pan or dish over low–medium heat and cook, stirring often, until the cooking liquid is slightly reduced and thickened. Serve the shanks with the sauce spooned over the top.

1 tablespoon gluten-free plain flour

sea salt and cracked black pepper

4 lamb shanks, french trimmed

2 tablespoons olive oil

1 onion, finely diced

1 carrot, finely diced

1 large stalk celery, trimmed and finely diced

2 cloves garlic, thinly sliced

small handful of rosemary leaves, roughly chopped

2 bay leaves

1 tablespoon gluten-free tomato paste (puree)

200 ml white wine

1 cup (250 ml) gluten-free chicken stock

SICILIAN MEATBALLS GRILLED *in* LEMON LEAVES

SERVES: 4

	PER SERVE
ENERGY (KJ/CAL)	1265/303
PROTEIN (G)	43.5
FAT (G)	13.5
SATURATED FAT (G)	5.5
CARBOHYDRATE (G)	1.5

2 teaspoons fennel seeds

small handful of marjoram leaves

2 cloves garlic, peeled

sea salt and cracked black pepper

300 g minced pork

300 g minced veal

50 g freshly grated pecorino

1 egg

40 small or 20 large pesticide-free lemon leaves

2 lemons, zest of 1 lemon finely grated, then both lemons halved

TOBIE I came across this little number in Sicily and absolutely loved it. Cooking with lemon leaves is so fantastic; the leaf gives flavour and also protects whatever it's enclosing from burning. You don't eat the lemon leaves though, so make sure you discard them after the cooking is done. You need to use pesticide-free lemon leaves and give them a good wipe with paper towel before using. Before you start shaping the meatballs into patties, cook just a marble-sized amount of the mixture to check the seasoning, then adjust as necessary. I always do this if I have time, so I know if they need more salt or pepper before it's too late.

Toast the fennel seeds in a dry frying pan over low–medium heat for a minute or so, until aromatic. Transfer to a mortar, add the marjoram, garlic and a pinch of salt and use the pestle to pound to a paste.

Put the pork, veal, pecorino, egg, lemon zest and marjoram mixture in a large bowl and use your hands to mix thoroughly. Season with pepper. Shape the mixture into 20 patties the size of golf balls, flattening them slightly as you go. Sandwich each patty between 2 lemon leaves or, if you are using larger leaves, wrap a leaf around each patty to enclose it. You may need to use toothpicks to secure the leaves.

Preheat a barbecue or grill plate on medium–high. When it is hot, place the lemon halves on it, flesh side down, and cook for 5 minutes, until the flesh side is quite dark in colour. Add the meatballs to the barbecue or grill plate and cook for 2 minutes on each side or until just cooked through.

Remove the lemon leaves from the meatballs and discard. Serve the meatballs with the beautiful juice of the grilled lemons squeezed over.

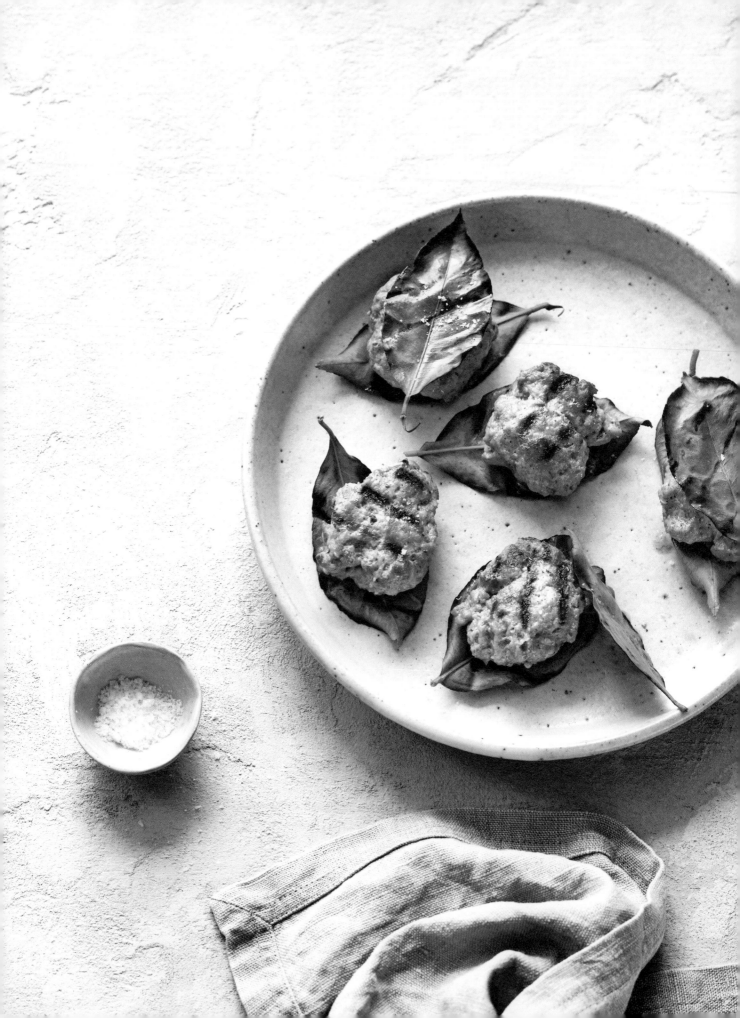

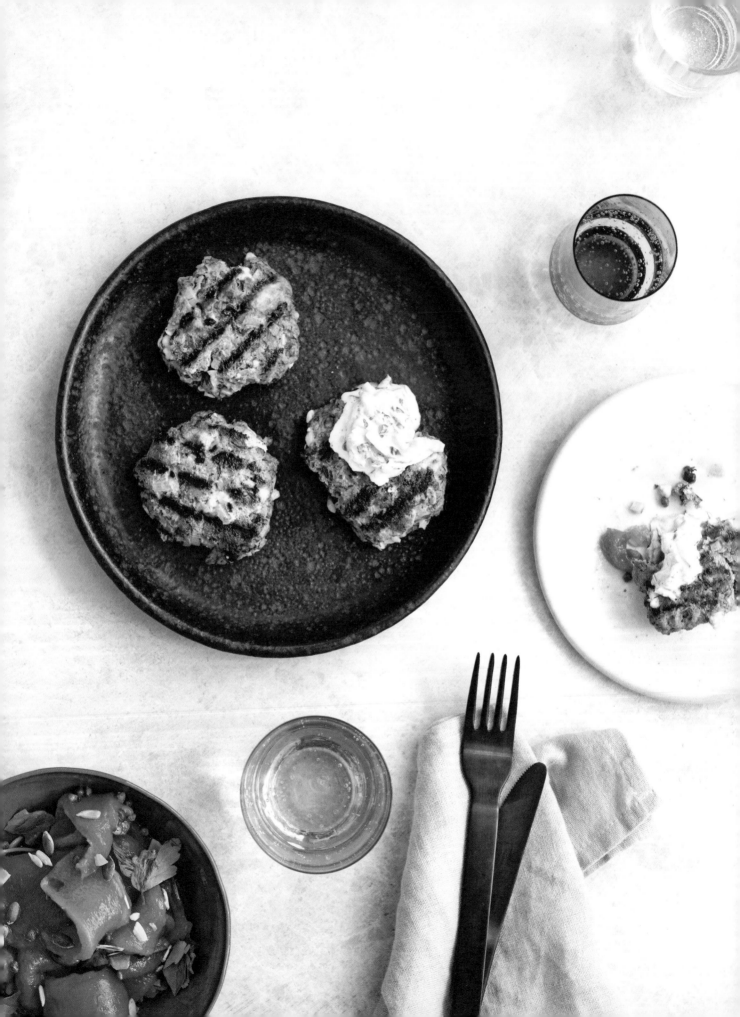

SPICED LAMB BURGERS
with TZATZIKI

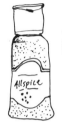
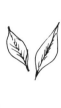

TOBIE I'll let you in on a little trick of mine. Whenever I make this recipe, I double or triple the quantities and then freeze the excess uncooked patties. It hardly takes any extra time and then I have a good stack of patties on hand that require no more effort than thawing and cooking. If you use bought tzatziki, check the label to make sure it's gluten free (homemade tzatziki is gluten-free by nature). This is delicious with the Roast capsicum with capers, seeds and nuts on page 113.

Heat the olive oil in a small frying pan over medium heat. Add the onion and garlic and cook, stirring often, for 2 minutes, until slightly softened but not coloured. Stir in the allspice, coriander, cumin, chilli flakes and mint and cook for a further minute. Take off the heat and set aside to cool.

Place the lamb in a large bowl and add the onion mixture, parsley, dill, egg, feta, salt and pepper. Use your hands to mix everything well. Shape the mixture into 4 patties, place on a tray and refrigerate for 10 minutes.

Preheat a grill plate on high. When it's hot, add the patties and cook for 3–4 minutes on each side or until just cooked through.

Serve the burgers with a dollop of tzatziki and a salad of your choice.

SERVES: 4

	PER SERVE
ENERGY (KJ/CAL)	1867/447
PROTEIN (G)	39.5
FAT (G)	28
SATURATED FAT (G)	11
CARBOHYDRATE (G)	8

2 tablespoons olive oil

¼ onion, finely diced

1 clove garlic, finely chopped

1 tablespoon ground allspice

2 teaspoons ground coriander

1 teaspoon ground cumin

½ teaspoon dried chilli flakes

1 tablespoon dried mint leaves

500 g minced lamb

small handful of flat-leaf parsley, roughly chopped

small handful of dill, roughly chopped

1 egg, lightly whisked

100 g reduced-fat feta cheese, crumbled

sea salt and cracked black pepper

Tzatziki (see page 188), to serve

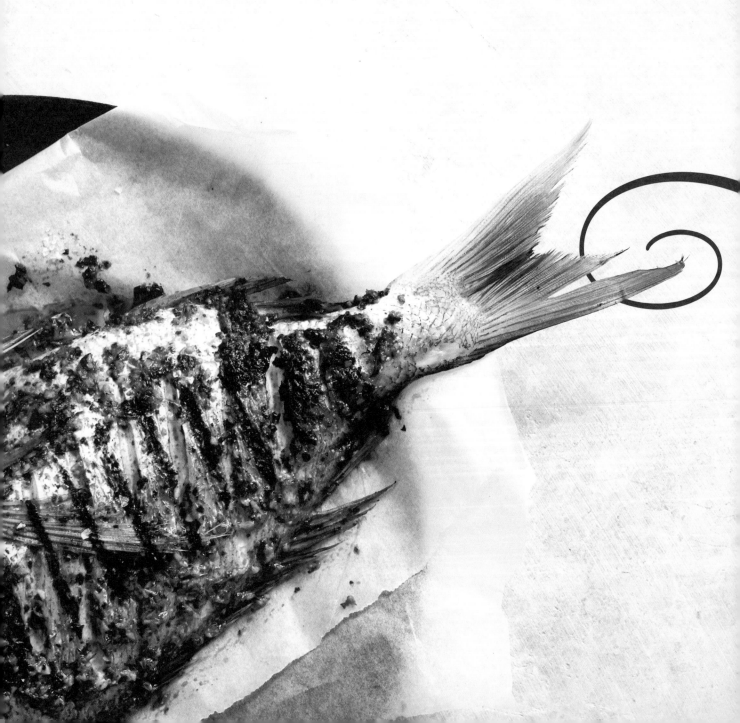

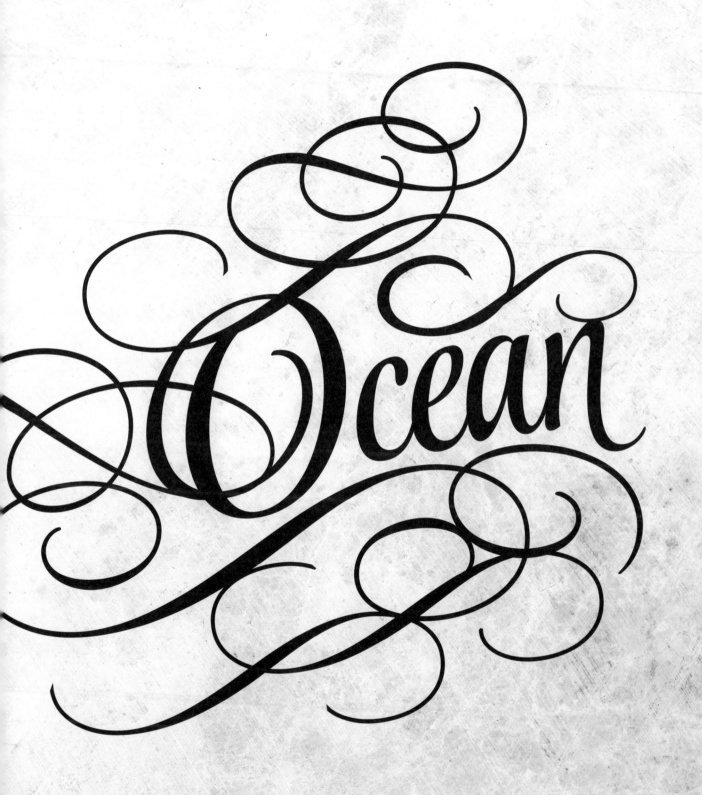

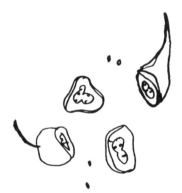

TUNA CARPACCIO
with CHILLI, CAPERS *and* MINT

SERVES: 4

	PER SERVE
ENERGY (KJ/CAL)	1044/250
PROTEIN (G)	37
FAT (G)	8.5
SATURATED FAT (G)	1.5
CARBOHYDRATE (G)	5

1 tablespoon thyme leaves, roughly chopped

sea salt and cracked black pepper

1 × 500 g piece of tuna

1½ tablespoons extra virgin olive oil, plus extra for drizzling

handful of mint leaves (about 20), finely chopped

1 red bird's-eye chilli, finely chopped

2 lemons, 1 halved and 1 quartered

1½ tablespoons salted baby capers, rinsed

handful of dill, roughly chopped

picked watercress, rocket or pea shoots, to serve

TOBIE Lots of the wonderful Italian dishes I've been cooking for so long work perfectly with our healthier way of eating. They feature big, bold flavours, using only the freshest ingredients, cooked simply. I've been making traditional tuna carpaccio since I was eighteen, but I was shown this seared version while working at The River Café in London and it's a winner. The slight charring of the thyme brings masses of flavour to the dish. Note that it's always preferable to ask your fishmonger for a middle piece of the loin and it should be in a single piece.

Preheat a barbecue or grill plate on high.

Scatter the thyme over a plate and add a good pinch of both salt and pepper. Rub the surface of the tuna with a teaspoon or two of olive oil and then roll it in the seasoned thyme, using your hands to push the thyme mixture onto the fish.

Put the mint and chilli in a small bowl and add just enough olive oil (about a tablespoon) to bring it together into a pesto-like consistency.

Place the lemon halves, flesh side down, on the hot barbecue or grill and cook for 5 minutes, until the flesh is quite dark in colour. Remove and set aside to cool for a few minutes, then squeeze the juice and any pulp that comes out into the mint mixture and stir to combine.

Barbecue or grill the tuna for 20–30 seconds on each side, then remove and leave to rest for a couple of minutes before slicing it as thinly as you can. (If any of your slices end up a bit thick, just put them between two layers of plastic film and flatten them lightly with a meat mallet or rolling pin.)

Arrange the tuna slices on serving plates or a large platter. Drizzle with the mint, chilli and grilled lemon dressing, then scatter over the capers, dill and cress or pea shoots. Season with a pinch of both salt and pepper, then finish with a little drizzle of olive oil and serve right away with the lemon quarters.

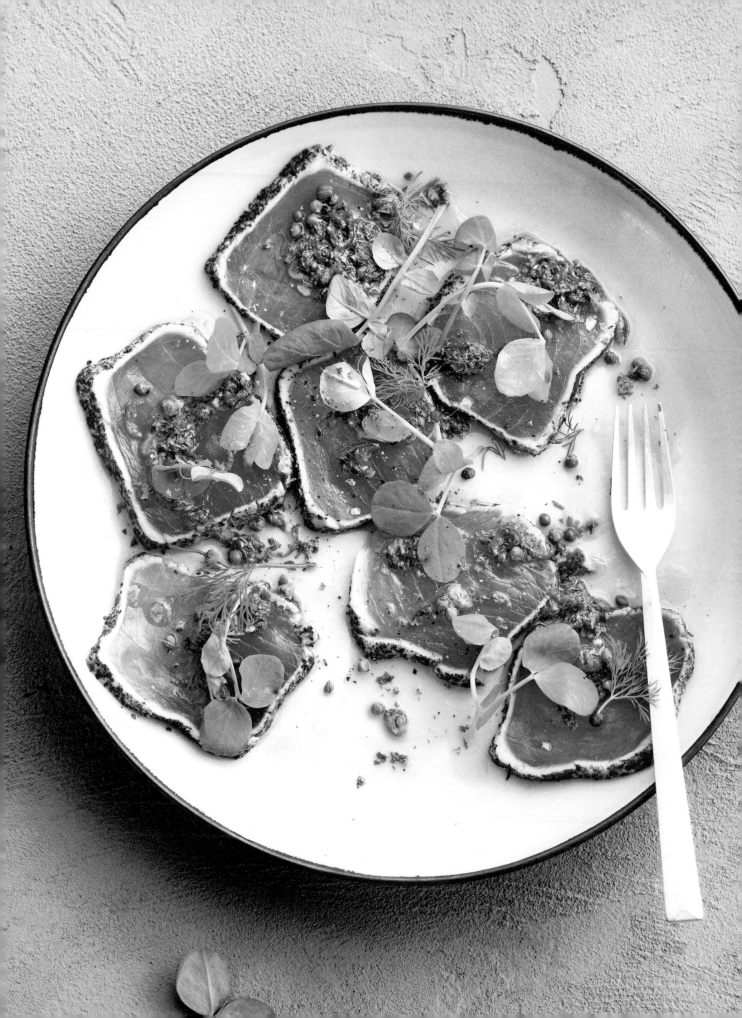

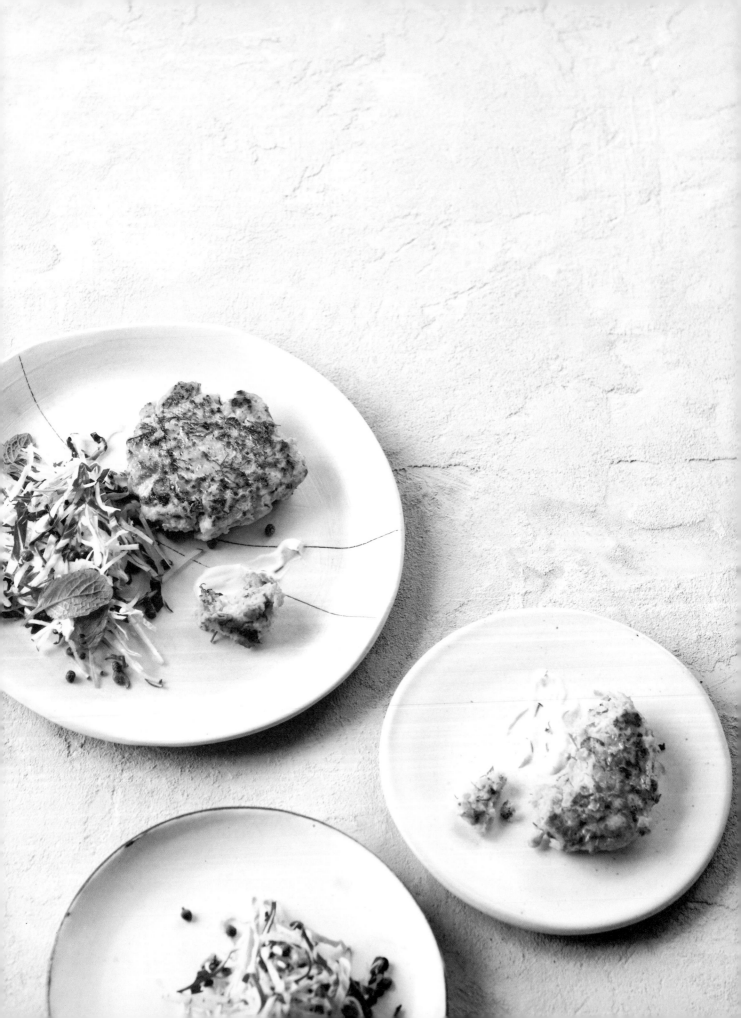

SWEET POTATO *and* SALMON FISHCAKES

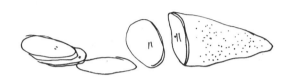

TOBIE Fishcakes generally contain potato and perhaps flour, and they're almost always deep-fried. As we don't use or do any of the above any more, I have been experimenting with other ingredients and methods, and got a fantastic result with this recipe. The almond meal helps bind everything together and of course the sweet potato is super low-carb. If you want a crispier crust on the fishcakes and don't mind a little more fat in the recipe, you can shallow-fry them using a couple of tablespoons of olive oil. If your fishmonger doesn't sell minced salmon, you can mince some fresh salmon yourself or finely chop it.

GEORGIA We are really big fans of chillies, both for their great flavour kick and also to help speed up the metabolism. If you wanted to add some chopped chilli to these fishcakes, add it to the mashed sweet potato with the other ingredients. We usually serve this with coleslaw (see the recipe on page 138) and minted low-fat plain Greek-style yoghurt.

SERVES: 4	
	PER SERVE
ENERGY (KJ/CAL)	1326/317
PROTEIN (G)	25.5
FAT (G)	17.5
SATURATED FAT (G)	3.5
CARBOHYDRATE (G)	13.5

Preheat the oven to 200°C. Line a baking tray with baking paper.

Place the sweet potato in a large saucepan, cover with cold water, add a good pinch of salt and bring to a simmer over medium–high heat. Reduce the heat and hold at a simmer for 15 minutes or until tender. Drain in a colander, refresh with cold water, then set aside to cool completely.

Transfer the sweet potato to a large bowl and mash using a potato masher. Add the salmon, almond meal, egg, orange zest, paprika, parsley, dill and a pinch each of salt and pepper. Mix until thoroughly combined.

Drizzle the olive oil over the lined tray. Shape the sweet potato mixture into 4 patties and place on the prepared tray. Bake the fishcakes for 5 minutes, then carefully turn them over and bake for another 5 minutes or until cooked through and golden.

---

300 g peeled and roughly chopped sweet potato

sea salt and cracked black pepper

300 g minced fresh salmon

3 teaspoons almond meal

1 egg, lightly whisked

finely grated zest of ¼ orange

1 teaspoon hot smoked paprika

small handful of flat-leaf parsley, finely chopped

small handful of dill, roughly chopped

1 tablespoon extra virgin olive oil

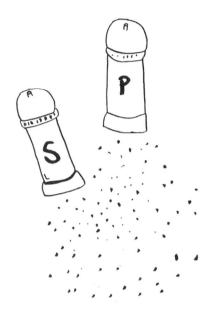

TRAY-BAKED FISH

This is the easiest way to cook fish that I know of and I want to include it here because so many people don't know how to cook fish and are scared to try. This recipe can be used for salmon, ocean trout, blue-eye trevalla, sea bass, bream, mackerel, mahi mahi, kingfish and barramundi, though the cooking time will vary depending on the size and density of the fillets used. Although many recipes for roasting fish fillets require them to be sealed in oil or another fat before going in the oven, this really isn't necessary. I like to use two larger fillets, but of course you can use four 180 g fillets if you prefer.

GEORGIA To be honest with you, I really only cook when Tobie is away, so although I know a lot about food and flavour, my technical abilities are pretty limited. This, however, is my kind of recipe. It comes out perfectly every time. You can use whatever herbs you have, but the woody ones hold up better in the oven.

SERVES: 4

	PER SERVE
ENERGY (KJ/CAL)	973/233
PROTEIN (G)	36.5
FAT (G)	9
SATURATED FAT (G)	2
CARBOHYDRATE (G)	1

2 × 360 g portions of fish, skin on

4 sprigs rosemary, halved

sea salt and cracked black pepper

2 lemons

2 teaspoons extra virgin olive oil

Preheat the oven to 220°C. Line a large baking tray with baking paper.

Place the fish on a chopping board and use a sharp knife to make 4 lengthways incisions into the skin of each portion, no more than 5 mm deep. Push a rosemary sprig into each. Season the fish generously with salt and pepper and squeeze over the juice of 1 lemon. Drizzle the oil over the lined tray and place the fish, flesh side down, on the prepared tray.

Bake the fish for 10–12 minutes, until the flesh flakes easily when tested with a fork, then remove from the oven and set aside for 1 minute to rest. Use a large sharp knife to cut each portion of fish in half, then cut the remaining lemon into quarters and serve.

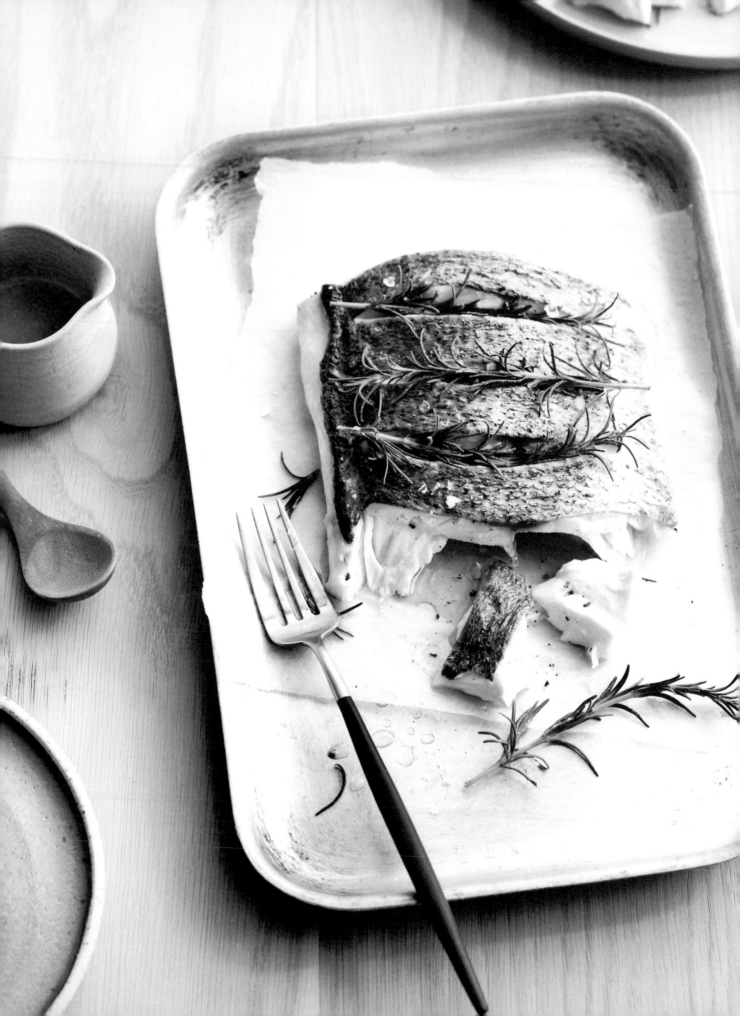

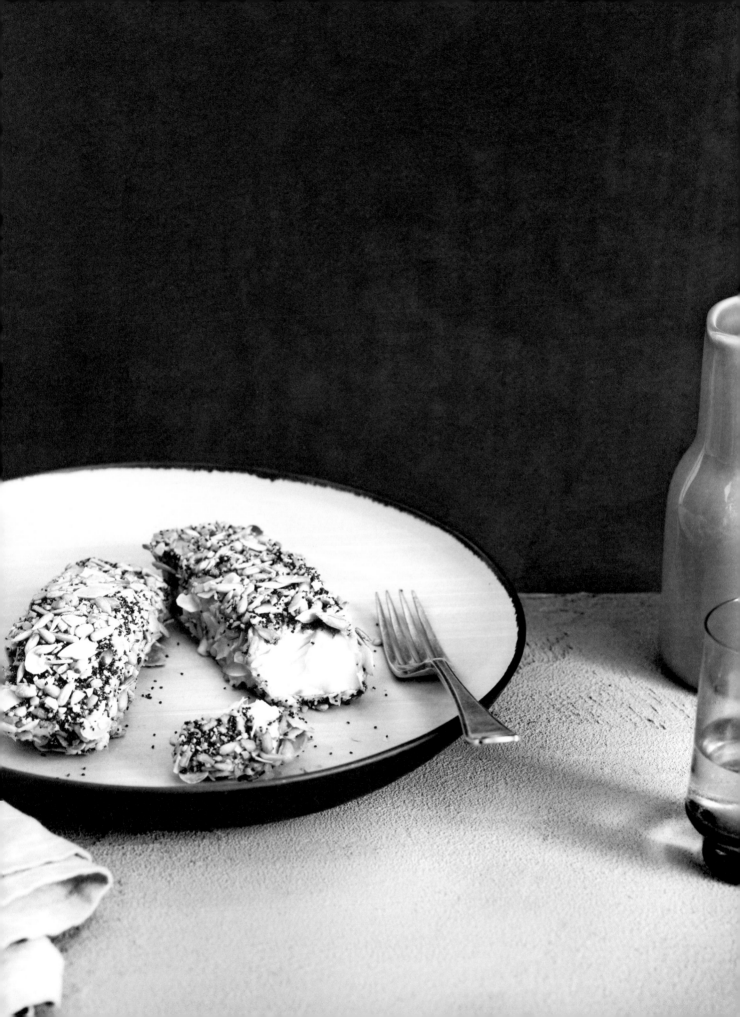

BLUE-EYE *with a* SEED *and* NUT CRUST

TOBIE I came across a recipe similar to this some years ago in Italy, however the fish was shallow-fried. I took inspiration from it and started playing with the concept of baking the fish and have had magnificent results. The combination of nuts and seeds I give here is my favourite, but I change it up depending on what's in the cupboard and I encourage you to do the same. If you have some Seed and nut mix (see page 190) on hand, feel free to use it instead. This type of crust works well on chicken fillets, too.

GEORGIA I don't eat meat, so we tend to consume a fair amount of seafood. When Tobie presented me with this dish, it blew me away. It's amazingly textural and somewhat reminiscent of fried fish, only healthy.

Preheat the oven to 200°C.

Put the almonds, pine nuts and sunflower seeds in a dry frying pan over medium heat and cook, stirring often, until toasted and aromatic. Place on a plate and sprinkle over the poppy seeds.

Crack the eggs into a shallow bowl and lightly whisk. Place the flour in a separate shallow bowl. Working one at a time, dust each fish fillet in the flour, then coat in the egg, allowing any excess to drip off. Place in the seed and nut mixture and use your hands to press it on so that both sides of each fillet are well coated.

Line a large baking tray with baking paper and drizzle with the olive oil. Place the fish on the prepared tray, allowing a little room between each fillet if possible. Bake the fish for 10–12 minutes, until the flesh flakes easily when tested with a fork.

Serve the fish immediately, with lemon halves or minted yoghurt.

SERVES: 4

	PER SERVE
ENERGY (KJ/CAL)	2750/658
PROTEIN (G)	48.5
FAT (G)	45
SATURATED FAT (G)	4
CARBOHYDRATE (G)	13

100 g flaked almonds

60 g pine nuts

80 g sunflower seed kernels

20 g black poppy seeds

2 eggs

½ cup (75 g) gluten-free plain flour

4 × 180 g skinless blue-eye trevalla fillets (or other firm white-fleshed fish fillets)

1 tablespoon extra virgin olive oil

lemon halves or minted low-fat plain Greek-style yoghurt, to serve

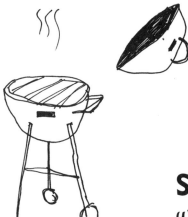

SMOKY BARBECUED SALMON
with PAPRIKA *and* CUMIN

SERVES: 4

	PER SERVE
ENERGY (KJ/CAL)	1682/402
PROTEIN (G)	38
FAT (G)	27
SATURATED FAT (G)	6
CARBOHYDRATE (G)	2

2 tablespoons hot smoked paprika

1 tablespoon ground cumin

2 tablespoons extra virgin olive oil

4 × 160 g salmon fillets, skin on, or a 640 g piece, skin on

rocket leaves, to serve

TOBIE Although this recipe is perfectly suited to salmon, you could use pretty well any type of fish. (The spice rub even works well on chicken.) I like to use a whole piece of fish, so if I'm cooking for four I ask my fishmonger for a piece of salmon that weighs approximately 640 g. It looks great and it's easier to keep the moisture in the flesh. Always ask them to pin-bone it for you, because doing it yourself with tweezers is quite fiddly work.

GEORGIA I love it when Tobie cooks fish on the barbecue, because it's such a healthy cooking method and doesn't leave the house smelling of fish. This is one of my all-time favourite dishes – it's simple, the ingredients are easy to find and it's so full of flavour. We often serve it when friends come over, paired with the Grilled zucchini with mint, feta and pine nuts on page 110.

Preheat the barbecue, grill plate or a chargrill pan on high.

Put the paprika, cumin and olive oil in a small bowl and stir to combine. Use a pastry brush or your fingers to brush or rub the spice mixture all over the salmon.

Place the salmon on the preheated barbecue, grill or pan, skin side up, and cook for 3 minutes, then flip over and cook for a further 4 minutes or until just cooked through and the flesh flakes easily when tested with a fork (the timing will depend upon the thickness of the fillets).

Remove from the heat and leave to rest for a few minutes before serving with some rocket alongside.

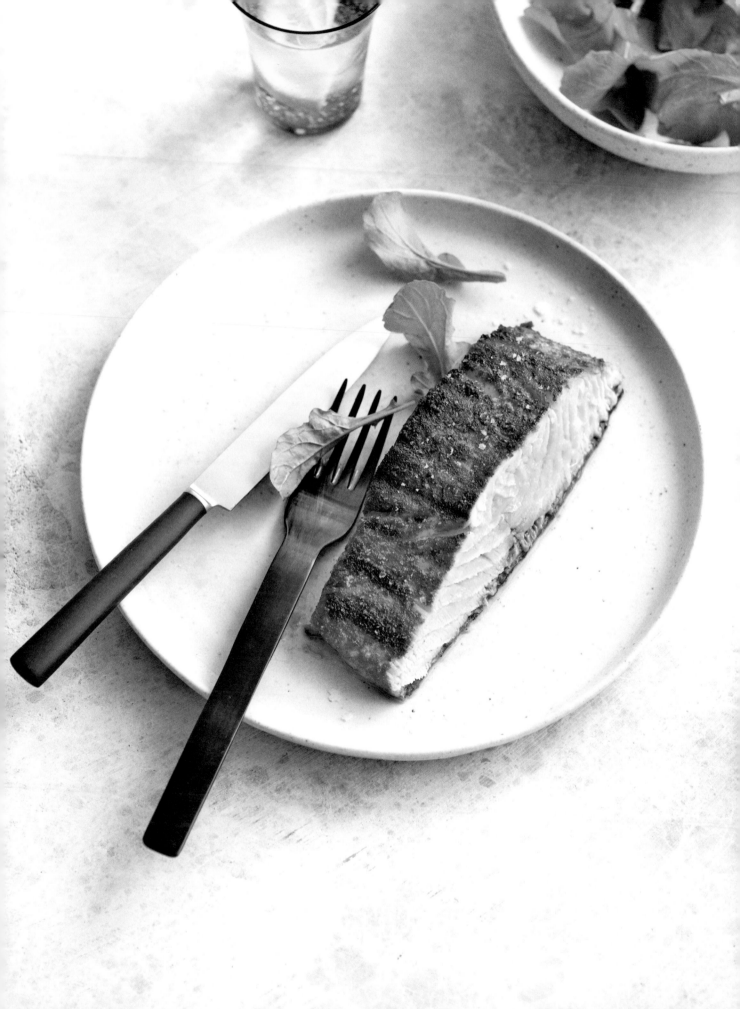

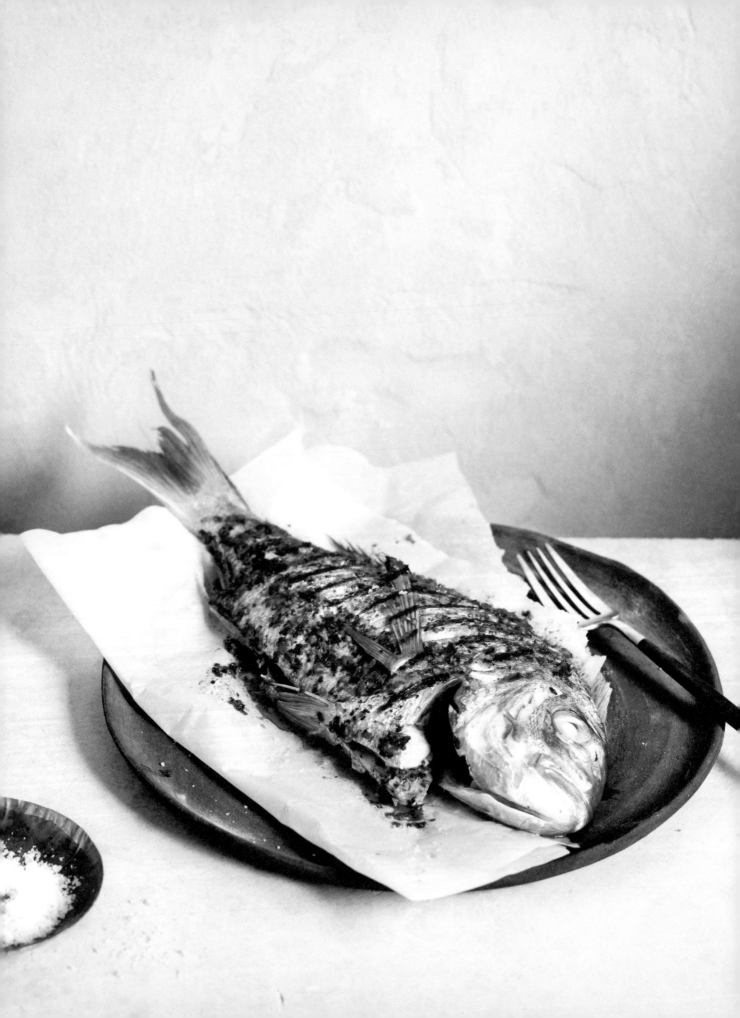

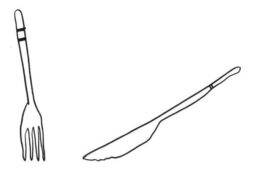

ROASTED WHOLE SNAPPER
with CHERMOULA

TOBIE I have been focused on Italian food for so many years that recipes such as this passed me by, but not any more. I always have chermoula in the fridge now. In this recipe I use a whole fish, but I also like to rub the chermoula over fish fillets and barbecue them. The result is awesome either way.

GEORGIA Using herbs and spices is the best way to impart flavour into a dish. Chermoula has become one of my favourite herb and spice pastes, and would work just as well on meat if you don't fancy fish.

Rub the chermoula all over the fish, including inside the cavity. Place on a plate, cover with plastic film and put in the fridge for at least 2 hours to marinate. Remove from the oven 20 minutes before cooking.

Preheat the oven to 200°C. Line a large baking tray with baking paper and brush with the olive oil.

Place the fish on the prepared tray and roast for 30–40 minutes or until it is just cooked through and the flesh flakes easily when tested with a fork. Serve right away.

SERVES: 4

	PER SERVE
ENERGY (KJ/CAL)	734/176
PROTEIN (G)	28
FAT (G)	7
SATURATED FAT (G)	1.5
CARBOHYDRATE (G)	0.5

2 tablespoons Chermoula (see page 187)

1 cleaned and gutted whole snapper (about 1.2 kg)

2 teaspoons extra virgin olive oil

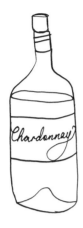

CLAMS *with* CHILLI, GARLIC, PARSLEY *and* WHITE WINE

SERVES: 4 AS A STARTER

	PER SERVE
ENERGY (KJ/CAL)	746/178
PROTEIN (G)	14
FAT (G)	12.5
SATURATED FAT (G)	2
CARBOHYDRATE (G)	1

1 kg clams (vongole)

2½ tablespoons extra virgin olive oil

4 cloves garlic, finely chopped

1–2 red bird's-eye chillies, thinly sliced

50 ml full-bodied white wine (such as chardonnay)

handful of flat-leaf parsley, roughly chopped

cracked black pepper

TOBIE When I was in Spain a few years ago, I was served a massive plate of clams cooked like this and it was just glorious. This is now a bit of a go-to dish for me when I have friends around. It's basically my spaghetti vongole, without the spaghetti. Clams often have some grit inside, so it's really important to soak them before cooking. When they're done, lift them out of the water using your hands so you don't bring any sand with you and place them in a clean bowl ready to be cooked. This goes beautifully with the Kale with chilli, garlic and lemon on page 102 – you can mop up the juices with the kale.

GEORGIA This is an absolute winner for dinner parties, because it looks fancy and is really quick to make. Just put the pan in the middle of the table and watch the clams disappear.

Place the clams in a large bowl, fill it with cold water and set aside for 30 minutes to 1 hour; they will spit out any sand during this time. Lift them out of the water using your hands, ensuring you leave any grit in the bottom of the bowl. Place the cleaned clams in a clean bowl or colander.

Heat the oil, garlic and chilli in a large heavy-based saucepan over medium heat. When the garlic starts to sizzle, stir with a wooden spoon and increase the heat to high. Add the clams and stir to distribute the garlic and chilli. Add the wine and pop the lid on the pan. Cook for 30 seconds, then lift the lid and check that the clams are starting to open. Cover again and cook until all the clams have opened, lifting the lid to see how they're progressing from time to time. Once all the clams have opened, fold through the parsley, season with pepper and serve right away.

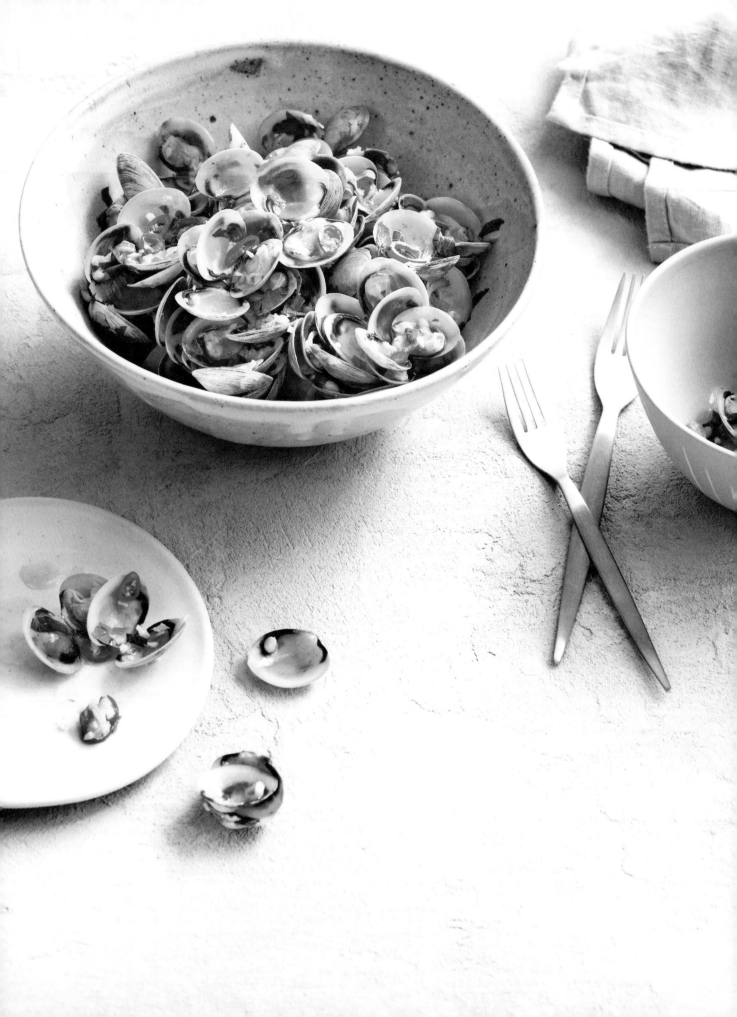

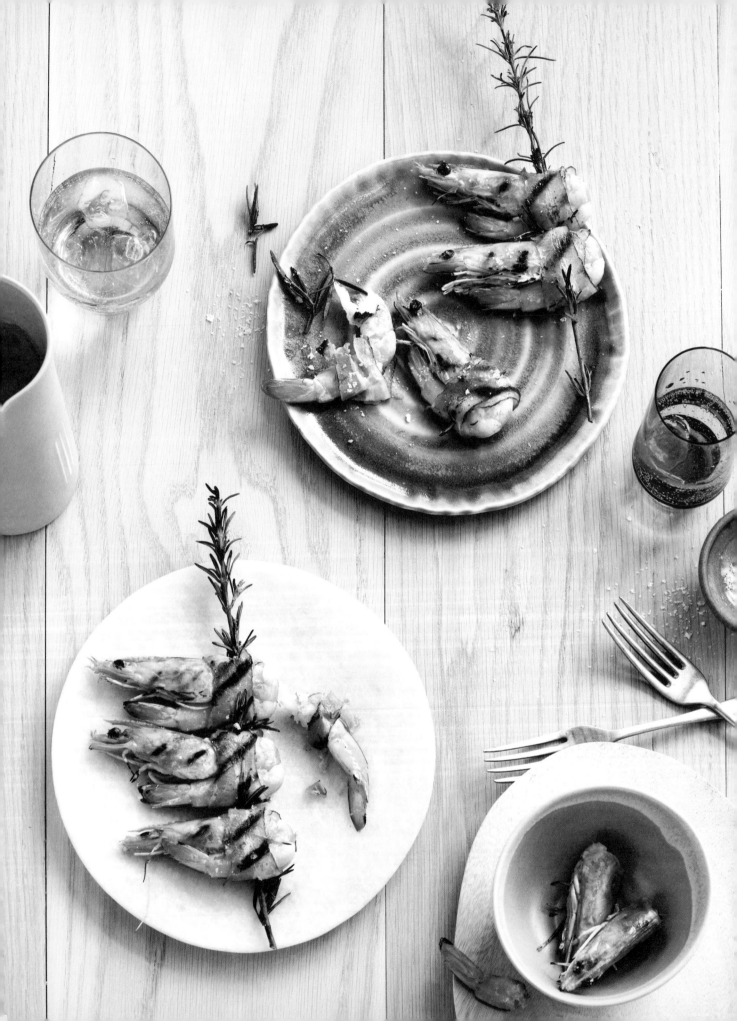

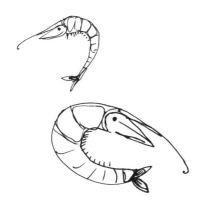

ROSEMARY SKEWERED PRAWNS *and* PANCETTA

TOBIE Georgia doesn't eat meat, but I have used pancetta in this recipe because it works so beautifully. The pancetta fat melts through the prawns as they cook, giving them loads of flavour. When I'm making these for Georgia I just leave the pancetta out, so of course you can do that too if you like. If you don't have a problem with gluten, you can add some torn ciabatta to the skewers. You need long, thick sprigs of rosemary to skewer the prawns, so if you grow it at home or know someone who does, cut them off the bush yourself. The sprigs you get at the supermarket are generally too soft to use in this way.

GEORGIA This dish is pure summer – perfect for a barbecue with friends, along with a couple of salads and a chilled glass of wine. So much better than chucking a few snags on the barbie!

Preheat a barbecue or grill plate on high.

Arrange the prawns so they're all curled up and wrap a piece of pancetta around each. Slide 3 wrapped prawns onto each rosemary sprig and season with pepper. Use a pastry brush to brush the wrapped prawns with a little olive oil and cook on the barbecue or grill for 3–4 minutes or until opaque.

Serve the prawns right away with the mustard and caper mayonnaise.

SERVES: 4

	PER SERVE
ENERGY (KJ/CAL)	1333/319
PROTEIN (G)	15.5
FAT (G)	28.5
SATURATED FAT (G)	5
CARBOHYDRATE (G)	1

4 large sprigs rosemary
(or 12 smaller ones)

12 large uncooked prawns, peeled and deveined, with heads and tails left intact

12 slices streaky flat pancetta

cracked black pepper

extra virgin olive oil, for brushing

Mustard and caper mayonnaise
(see page 193), to serve

GRILLED SEAFOOD *with* MARJORAM SALMORIGLIO

SERVES: 4

	PER SERVE
ENERGY (KJ/CAL)	1566/375
PROTEIN (G)	35
FAT (G)	25
SATURATED FAT (G)	4
CARBOHYDRATE (G)	2

1 medium squid (about 200 g), cleaned and gutted

400 g fillet white-fleshed fish (such as blue-eye), cut into 4 equal pieces

4 large uncooked prawns, peeled and deveined, with heads left intact

sea salt and cracked black pepper

extra virgin olive oil, for drizzling and brushing

1 quantity Marjoram salmoriglio (see page 182)

300 g clams or pipis, washed to remove any grit (see page 84)

2 lemons, halved

TOBIE I'd never really grilled shellfish much in the past, but I tried it at home last summer on my little kettle barbecue and quickly learnt that it's a good idea to put a fairly fine wire rack on the barbecue so they don't fall through. Once I had that sorted it was all go, a perfect summer night's dish. Here, I put the salmoriglio in a bowl and when each type of seafood is cooked it goes straight from the barbie to the bowl – any juices that come out of it mingle with the salmoriglio giving a really beautiful result.

Preheat a barbecue or grill plate on high and place a fine wire rack on it.

Cut the tentacles off the squid and reserve, then cut open the hood, score in a criss-cross pattern and cut into random shapes. Place the fish, prawns and squid, including the tentacles, on a plate and season with salt and pepper, then drizzle with a little olive oil (no more than 1 tablespoon). Put the salmoriglio in a large bowl and keep it close at hand.

Brush the barbecue or grill with a little olive oil, then carefully place the fish pieces on it, side by side. Cook for 2 minutes, then turn the fish and add the clams or pipis (you can put them straight on the hot plate or grill), followed by the prawns and the lemon halves, flesh side down. When the fish is cooked (about 2 minutes more – this will vary depending on the size of your fillets), carefully transfer it to the bowl with the salmoriglio.

When the prawns are golden underneath, turn them and cook the other side. When the lemons have darkened underneath, remove and set aside. As the clams or pipis start to open, remove them immediately using tongs and add to the salmoriglio. When the prawns are cooked, add them too.

Lastly, put the squid pieces and tentacles on the hot barbecue or grill and cook for about a minute on each side, until opaque, then add to the bowl.

Carefully toss the seafood together so that everything is coated with the salmoriglio. Arrange the seafood on a large platter or serving plates and serve right away with the grilled lemon.

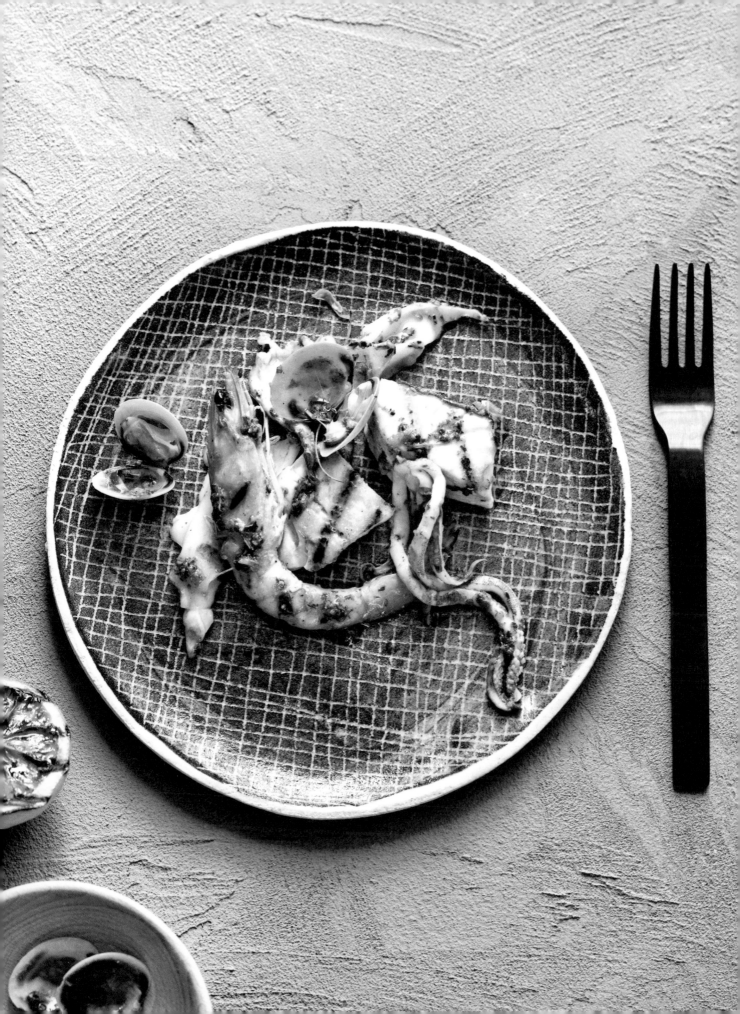

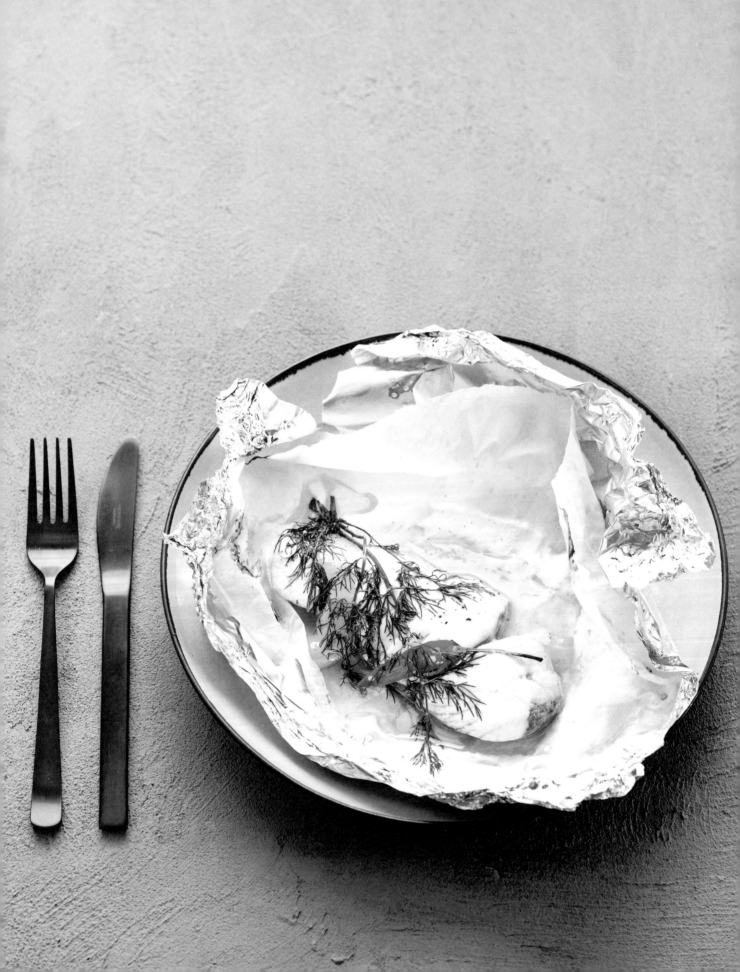

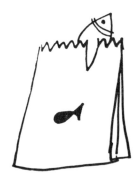

BLUE-EYE BAKED *in* a BAG

TOBIE Baking fish in a bag or parcel is nothing new and for good reason – it's an incredibly easy and effective way to cook fish. One of my favourite aspects of this method is that you can make up the bags ahead of time, then they're ready to cook whenever you are. What's great about it in terms of flavour is that everything is trapped in the bag, so any ingredients you add will directly enhance the fish. I like to put white wine in there, generally a full-bodied variety such as chardonnay, because it makes a beautiful saucy liquid to spoon over the cooked fish. Serve this with some Sweet potato mash (see page 129) and sliced avocado.

GEORGIA I always have this on high rotation when Tobie is away. It's simple, takes very little time to prepare and tastes delicious.

Preheat the oven to 200°C.

Tear off 4 pieces of foil, each about 30 cm long, then 4 pieces of baking paper, each about 25 cm long. Lay the pieces of foil out on your benchtop, then put a piece of baking paper on the centre of each.

Combine the wine, olive oil, lemon zest, dill, chilli, if using, and a good pinch of both salt and pepper in a large bowl. Stir to combine, then carefully add the fish fillets and turn them to coat with the marinade.

Place a fish fillet on each piece of paper, just off-centre. Use your fingers to fold up the edges of the paper and foil so they are secure and firm, leaving one side slightly open, then carefully distribute any remaining marinade among them. Close up all the parcels and place them on a large baking tray, leaving a little room between each if possible. Bake for 15–20 minutes or until the fish flakes easily when tested with a fork. Remove from the oven and leave to sit for a couple of minutes.

Carefully transfer the bags to serving plates and open them at the table (take care as there will be a build-up of steam inside).

SERVES: 4

	PER SERVE
ENERGY (KJ/CAL)	1003/240
PROTEIN (G)	32.5
FAT (G)	10.5
SATURATED FAT (G)	1.5
CARBOHYDRATE (G)	0.5

100 ml white wine

2 tablespoons extra virgin olive oil

long strips of zest from 1 lemon

small handful of dill sprigs

2 red bird's-eye chillies, halved lengthways (optional)

sea salt and cracked black pepper

4 × 180 g skinless blue-eye trevalla fillets

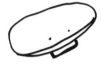

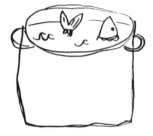

FISH *with* CAPERS, OLIVES *and* CHERRY TOMATOES

SERVES: 4

	PER SERVE
ENERGY (KJ/CAL)	1437/344
PROTEIN (G)	35.5
FAT (G)	18.5
SATURATED FAT (G)	2.5
CARBOHYDRATE (G)	4.5

400 g cherry tomatoes

2 tablespoons extra virgin olive oil, plus extra for drizzling

100 g black olives, pitted

2 tablespoons salted baby capers, rinsed

2 cloves garlic, thinly sliced

4 anchovy fillets

1 red bird's-eye chilli, finely chopped (optional)

100 ml white wine

4 × 180 g white fish fillets, skin on (such as blue-eye trevalla), each sliced into three even pieces

sea salt and cracked black pepper

good handful of flat-leaf parsley, roughly chopped

good handful of basil leaves, roughly torn

TOBIE This little recipe has come about from years of making *brodetto di mare*, the famous seafood stew of Sicily. What's so fabulous about this dish is that the cooking method, which is a combination of poaching and steaming, requires minimal oil and produces a really tender, flavoursome result. A full-bodied white wine, such as chardonnay, works best here.

Halve the cherry tomatoes and, holding them over a fine-meshed sieve set over a bowl, squeeze them to remove most of the seeds. Reserve the juice in the bowl with the tomato halves, and discard the seeds.

Heat the olive oil in a large heavy-based saucepan or deep frying pan over low–medium heat. Add the olives, capers, garlic, anchovies and chilli, if using, and cook gently for a couple of minutes to soften the garlic and infuse the flavours through the oil.

Add the tomato halves and juice and increase the heat to medium–high. Cook, stirring, for 1 minute, then add the wine. Carefully place the fish in the pan, partially cover with a lid and reduce the heat to low–medium. The fish should take 11–12 minutes to cook, though this will depend upon the size and shape of the fillets. (The fish is cooked when the flesh flakes easily when tested with a fork.) Remove the pan from the heat, taste the sauce and season with salt and pepper as needed. (I normally add a good pinch of both.) Scatter the herbs over the fish.

Use a spatula to divide the fish among serving plates, then spoon over the sauce. Finish with a drizzle of olive oil and some cracked black pepper.

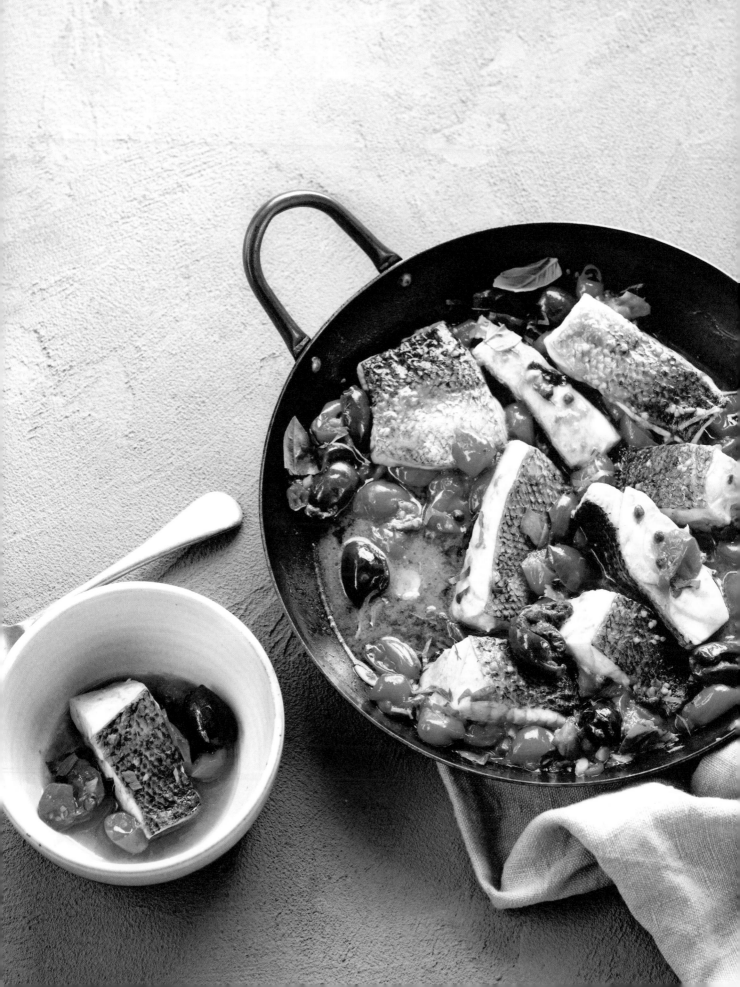

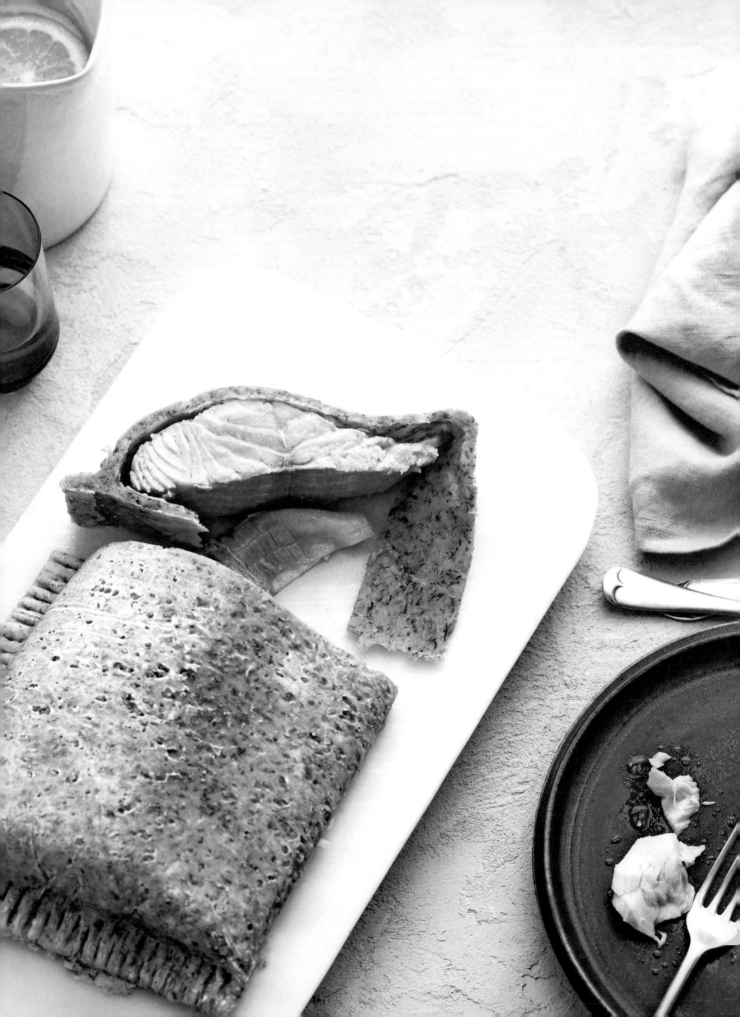

SALMON BAKED in SALTED DOUGH

TOBIE This may look difficult, but I promise it's not. Old cooking techniques like this are generally straightforward and proven to work – they wouldn't still be around otherwise! I use both a food processor and a stand mixer here. The food processor is more for aesthetic reasons and can be skipped if you want (just chop the herbs instead). The stand mixer is important though, because the rock salt is sharp, which makes mixing the dough by hand rather painful. Gluten-free flours differ between brands, so you may find you need to add a little more flour or water to get the dough right – it should have a slightly wet consistency.

GEORGIA I love serving this when we have people over – it always blows them away because it looks so beautiful and intriguing. The fish inside is so tender it just about melts in your mouth. This is my idea of heaven on a plate.

Place the salt, parsley and dill in a food processor and pulse briefly until the salt is green. Transfer to a stand mixer and add the flour, egg white and ⅓ cup (80 ml) water and use a dough hook to mix on low speed until the mixture comes together into a slightly wet dough. Add a little extra flour or water if required to get the right consistency. Wrap in plastic film and leave to rest for at least 1 hour before using.

Preheat the oven to 220°C.

Roll the dough out on a long sheet of baking paper to a 5 mm thickness. What you need is a rectangular shape large enough to encase the fish – if your dough is an odd shape, break off pieces and then press them on where they're needed to form a rectangle.

Place the salmon on one side of the dough and use a pastry brush to brush with the olive oil. Carefully fold the dough over the top so that the fish is enclosed. Use your fingers to push the dough down around the fish to make a neat seal. Use a small sharp knife to trim any excess dough. If the dough breaks at all, just pinch it back together or use a spare piece of dough to cover the crack.

Carefully lift the dough parcel, still on the baking paper, onto the lined tray and bake for 12 minutes. Remove from the oven and set aside for 2–3 minutes to rest. Carefully transfer to a platter and take to the table. Cut into the dough around the perimeter of the salmon and lift off the top of the dough. Slice the salmon into portions and serve. Discard the dough.

SERVES: 4

	PER SERVE
ENERGY (KJ/CAL)	1852/443
PROTEIN (G)	54
FAT (G)	25
SATURATED FAT (G)	6.5
CARBOHYDRATE (G)	0

250 g rock salt

small handful of flat-leaf parsley

small handful of dill

1⅓ cups (170 g) gluten-free plain flour

1 egg white

800 g salmon fillet (preferably one piece), pin-boned

1 teaspoon extra virgin olive oil

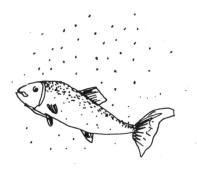

CRISPY-SKIN SALMON *with* DILL

SERVES: 4

	PER SERVE
ENERGY (KJ/CAL)	1556/372
PROTEIN (G)	44
FAT (G)	21.5
SATURATED FAT (G)	5.5
CARBOHYDRATE (G)	0

4 × 180 g salmon fillets, skin on and pin-boned

sea salt and cracked black pepper

small handful of dill, roughly chopped

extra virgin olive oil, for drizzling

lemon wedges, to serve

TOBIE The combination of salmon and dill needs no introduction. But what's special about this dish is that it's simple, quick to cook and tastes great – it's a regular at our place. While the barbie is heating up (ours uses coal so this takes a little while), I get the salmon in the marinade and make a salad or vegetable dish of some sort. The timing always works perfectly for me.

Place the salmon fillets on a chopping board, flesh side down, and use a sharp knife to make three lengthways incisions into the skin of each, about 5 mm deep.

Put the salmon fillets on a large plate and season with salt and pepper, then scatter over the dill and drizzle with olive oil. Turn the fillets over and use your hands to press the dill mixture all over the salmon, then cover with plastic film and set aside for about 20 minutes to marinate.

Preheat the barbecue, grill plate or chargrill pan on medium–high.

Cook the salmon, skin side down, on the hot barbecue or grill for 2–3 minutes, then turn and cook for a further 2–3 minutes or until the flesh flakes easily when tested with a fork. Remove from the heat and leave to rest for a few minutes before serving with lemon wedges.

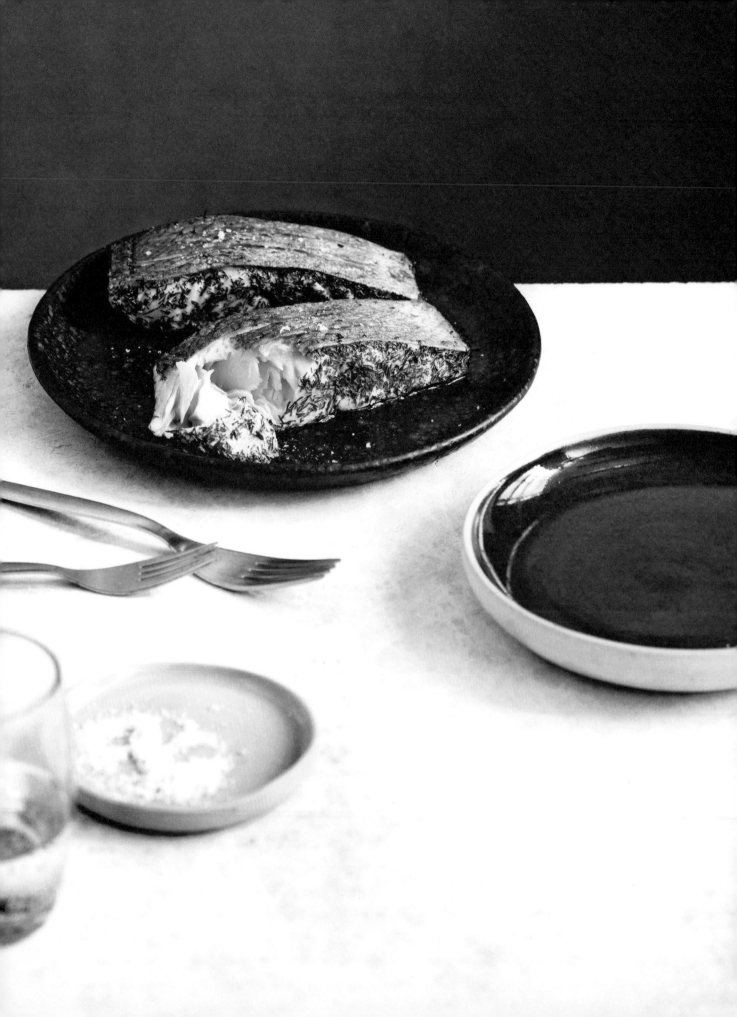

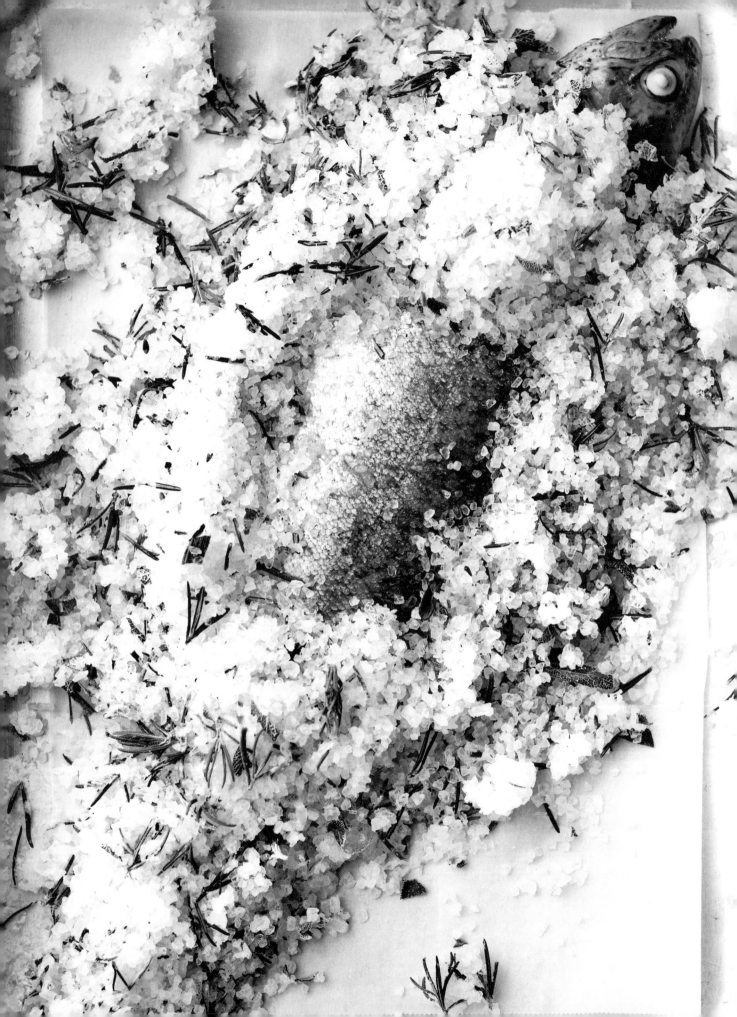

RAINBOW TROUT BAKED in SALT

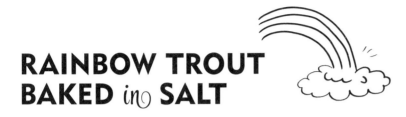

Before you turn the page thinking this looks a little too cheffy for you, please hear me out. I promise this recipe is really, really easy and just happens to look pretty fancy. It's an age-old technique and the flavour and texture it gives is unbelievable.

It's true you can only use the rock salt once, but it's not expensive. And a whole trout is relatively cheap, so all up it's probably cheaper than buying two salmon fillets. I like to throw a few herbs through the salt, usually whatever happens to be in the fridge, and although you don't have to do this it does add extra flavour. As with a few of the dishes in this chapter, you could use other fish here (whole or a single portion), though they may need more or less cooking time. If the fennel stalks on your bulb are rather short, use a few (you want about two or three 5 cm pieces all up).

Preheat the oven to 200°C. Line a large baking tray with baking paper.

Pat the fish with paper towel to remove any moisture, then place on a chopping board. Use a sharp knife to make 3 diagonal incisions, about 1–2 mm deep, on each side of the fish. Season the fish cavity generously with pepper, then stuff with the lemon slices, fennel, if using, and parsley.

Put the salt, herbs and 2 teaspoons water in a medium bowl and mix with your hands; the mixture should resemble wet sand. Scatter a quarter of the mixture over the baking paper to make a thin layer. Place the fish on top of the salt and then spread the remaining salt out over the top of the fish, using your hands to pat it down so it covers the fish snugly. Don't worry if the head and tail aren't covered – the edible part of the fish is the most important part.

Bake the fish for 20 minutes, then remove from the oven and rest for 5 minutes before removing the salt. Carefully transfer the fish to a platter and serve right away or place it on a chopping board, remove the head and then use a spatula to remove the flesh from the bones. Serve the fish with a light drizzle of extra virgin olive oil.

SERVES: 2

	PER SERVE
ENERGY (KJ/CAL)	1100/263
PROTEIN (G)	31
FAT (G)	15.5
SATURATED FAT (G)	4.5
CARBOHYDRATE (G)	0

1 whole rainbow trout, cleaned and gutted (about 450 g)

cracked black pepper

½ lemon, cut into three slices

1 fennel stalk, cut into 5 cm lengths (optional)

1–2 sprigs flat-leaf parsley

800 g rock salt

small handful of woody herbs (such as rosemary or sage), roughly chopped

extra virgin olive oil, for drizzling

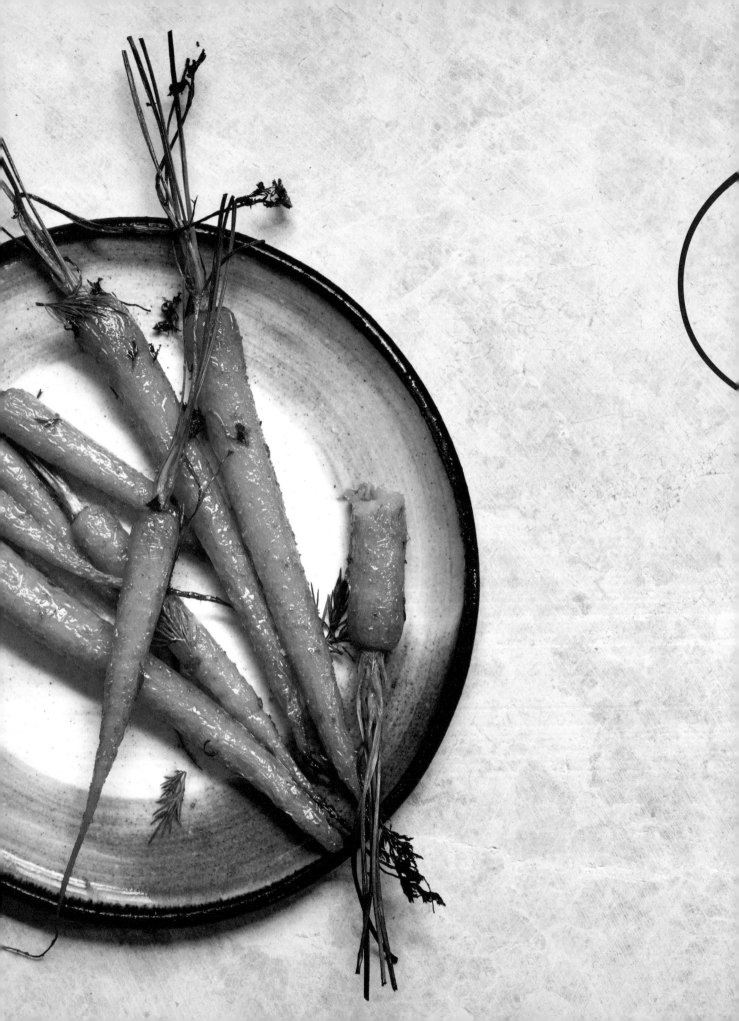

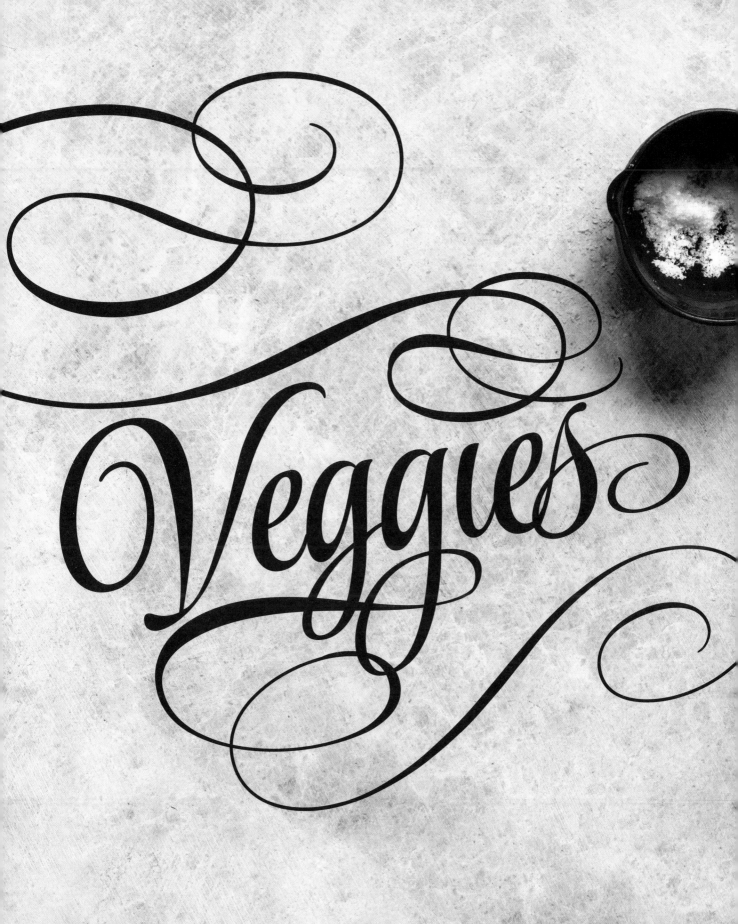

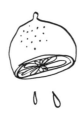

KALE *with* CHILLI, GARLIC *and* LEMON

SERVES: 4 AS A SIDE

	PER SERVE
ENERGY (KJ/CAL)	234/56
PROTEIN (G)	1
FAT (G)	4.5
SATURATED FAT (G)	0.5
CARBOHYDRATE (G)	2

1 bunch curly kale, stalks trimmed

1 tablespoon extra virgin olive oil

1 clove garlic, thinly sliced

6 anchovy fillets (optional)

1 small red chilli, finely chopped (optional)

juice of ½ lemon

sea salt and cracked black pepper

TOBIE Like most vegetables, the nutrients in kale are best retained when it's not cooked in boiling water. Here, I saute it to hold on to as many nutrients as possible. Kale has a very tough stalk that is not easy to digest, so it is best to trim the stalks off just below the leaves (you can keep them for juicing if you like).

GEORGIA The list of kale's nutritional values goes on and on, but in short this vegetable is incredibly good for you. We started eating it because we had heard it's so nutritious, but what really won us over was its flavour and versatility.

Place a few kale leaves on top of each other and slice into thick strips. Repeat with the remaining kale.

Heat the olive oil, garlic and anchovies and chilli, if using, in a large heavy-based saucepan over low–medium heat. When the garlic starts to sizzle, add the kale and 1 tablespoon of water and move the kale around the pan with a wooden spoon or tongs for 5 minutes or until it starts to wilt.

Season the kale with the lemon juice, salt and pepper – remembering that if you're using anchovies they will add salt, too. Serve immediately.

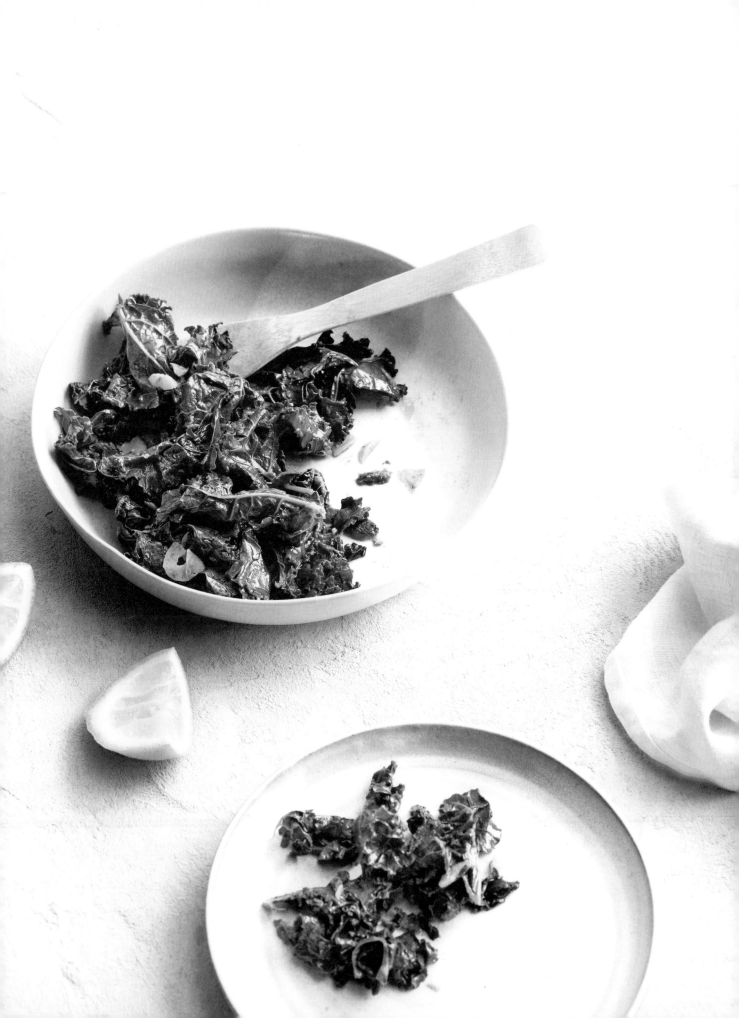

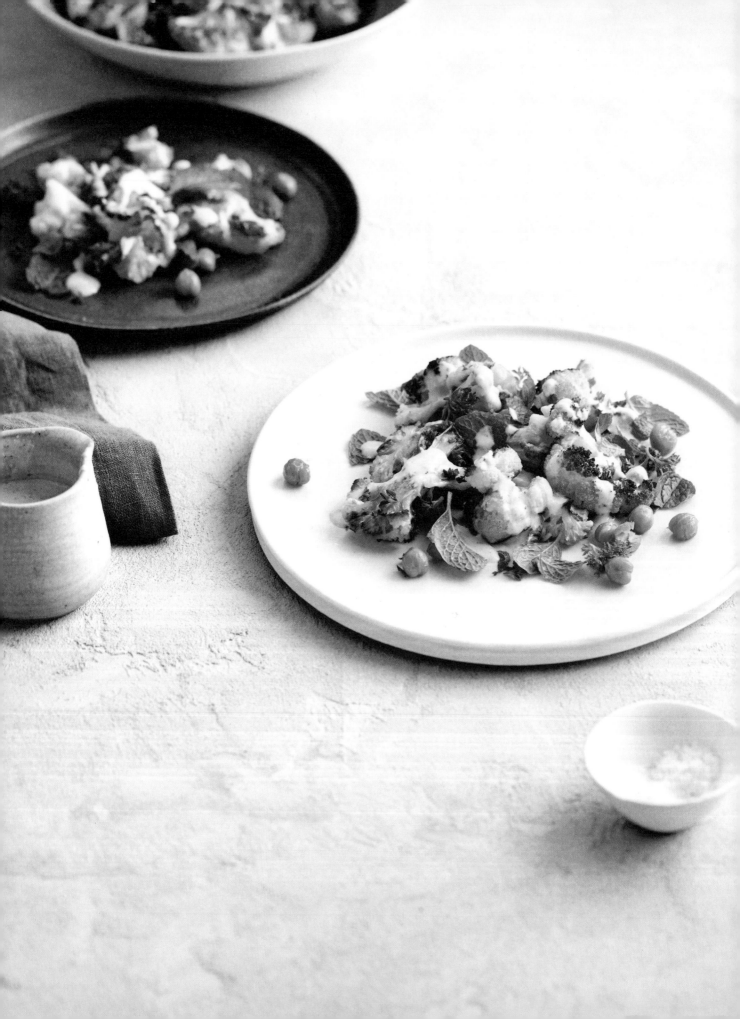

ROAST CAULIFLOWER *with* CHICKPEAS

TOBIE This is such a simple and tasty dish, with a great combination of flavours and textures. I usually get the cauliflower and chickpeas in the oven, then go off and cook up a piece of fish or meat – by the time that's done, all I need to do is come back and combine all the ingredients. Too easy! (I usually make a double quantity, too, to take care of lunch for a couple of days.)

GEORGIA If you haven't tried roasting cauliflower before, please give this a go. It develops a delicious nutty flavour and gets a little crispy on the edges. This dish works really well as a side dish instead of using potatoes. Note that flaxseed oil needs to be kept in the fridge to prevent it turning rancid and it shouldn't be heated as this destroys its nutritional value.

Preheat the oven to 180°C. Line 2 large baking trays with baking paper.

Use a small, sharp knife to remove the florets from the cauliflower; discard the core. Place the florets in a large bowl and season with 1 tablespoon of the olive oil, a good pinch of both salt and pepper and the chilli flakes, if using. Spread over a lined tray and roast for 30–40 minutes or until the cauliflower is quite dark around the edges and becoming crisp. Remove from the oven and leave to cool.

Meanwhile, scatter the chickpeas and garlic cloves over the other lined tray. Drizzle with the remaining 2 teaspoons of olive oil and jiggle the tray to combine. Roast for 20 minutes or until golden. Remove from the oven and leave to cool.

Squeeze the roasted garlic flesh into a bowl; discard the skins. Use a fork to mash the garlic, then add the cayenne pepper, tahini, yoghurt, extra virgin olive oil or flaxseed oil, lemon juice and water and stir to combine. Have a taste and adjust the seasoning as necessary.

Divide the cauliflower and chickpeas among serving plates, drizzle with the dressing and scatter the mint and parsley over the top. Serve.

SERVES: 4 AS A SIDE

	PER SERVE
ENERGY (KJ/CAL)	1009/241
PROTEIN (G)	7.5
FAT (G)	16.5
SATURATED FAT (G)	3
CARBOHYDRATE (G)	12.5

½ large cauliflower

1½ tablespoons extra virgin olive oil

sea salt and cracked black pepper

1 teaspoon dried chilli flakes (optional)

400 g tin chickpeas, rinsed and drained

2 cloves garlic, unpeeled

1 teaspoon cayenne pepper

1 tablespoon gluten-free hulled tahini

2 tablespoons low-fat plain Greek-style yoghurt

1 tablespoon extra virgin olive oil or flaxseed oil

juice of 1 lemon

2 tablespoons warm water

good handful of mint leaves, torn

good handful of continental parsley, roughly chopped

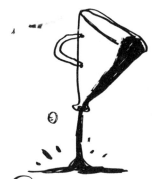

SPINACH with PINE NUTS, GARLIC and BALSAMIC

SERVES: 4 AS A SIDE

	PER SERVE
ENERGY (KJ/CAL)	405/97
PROTEIN (G)	4
FAT (G)	7.5
SATURATED FAT (G)	1
CARBOHYDRATE (G)	2

500 g baby spinach leaves, washed twice

1 tablespoon olive oil

1 small red onion, thinly sliced

1 large clove garlic, finely chopped

1 fresh red chilli, seeded and thinly sliced (optional)

1 tablespoon pine nuts

1 tablespoon balsamic vinegar

sea salt and cracked black pepper

TOBIE | I've been making this dish since I was a kid working at Melbourne's Caffé e Cucina, and I'll be making it for many more years to come. It's got it all – spinach (the food of the gods!), sweet balsamic, caramelised onion and garlic, and crunchy pine nuts. Bliss. If you want to hold onto more of the nutrients from the spinach, simply wilt it in the pan with the onions, rather than blanching it. Use the best-quality balsamic vinegar you can afford, as it's a key ingredient here.

Blanch the baby spinach in a saucepan of boiling salted water for 30 seconds or until wilted. Drain in a fine-meshed sieve and refresh under cold running water. Cool to room temperature, then squeeze out as much water as you can. Set aside until needed. Wipe down the pan with paper towel.

Heat the olive oil in the saucepan over low heat. Add the onion, garlic and chilli, if using, and cook, stirring often, for 10 minutes or until the onion is soft and translucent. Add the pine nuts, increase the heat to medium and cook, stirring, until they just begin to brown.

Add the blanched spinach to the pan and cook, stirring, for 1 minute before adding the balsamic vinegar. Stir to combine, then season with salt and pepper and serve.

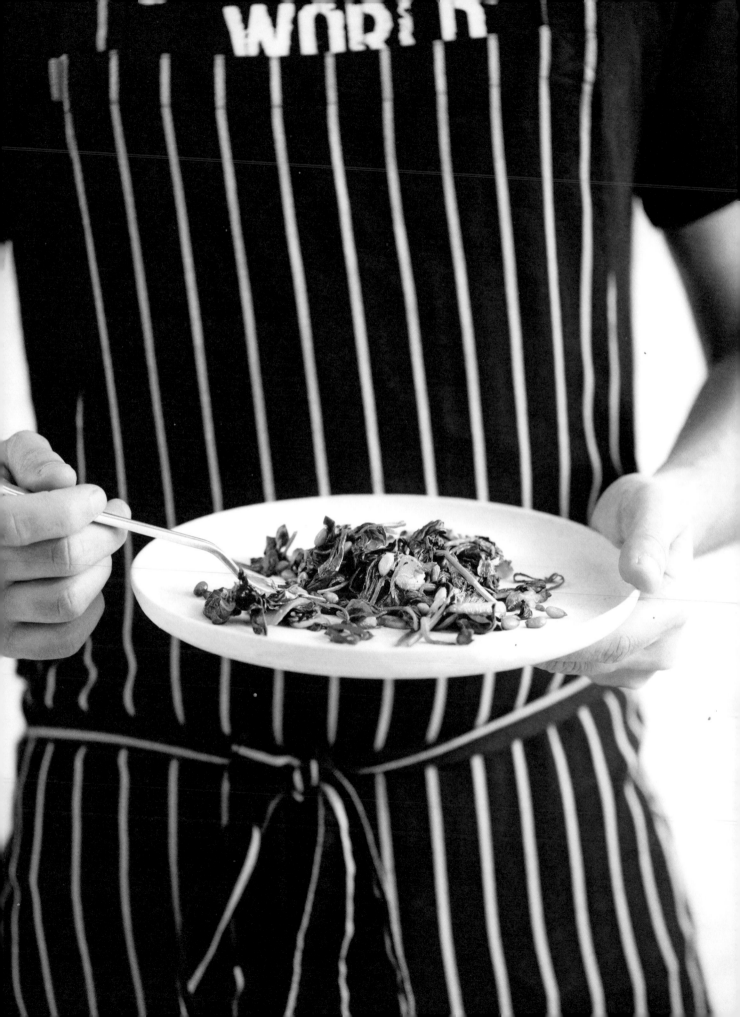

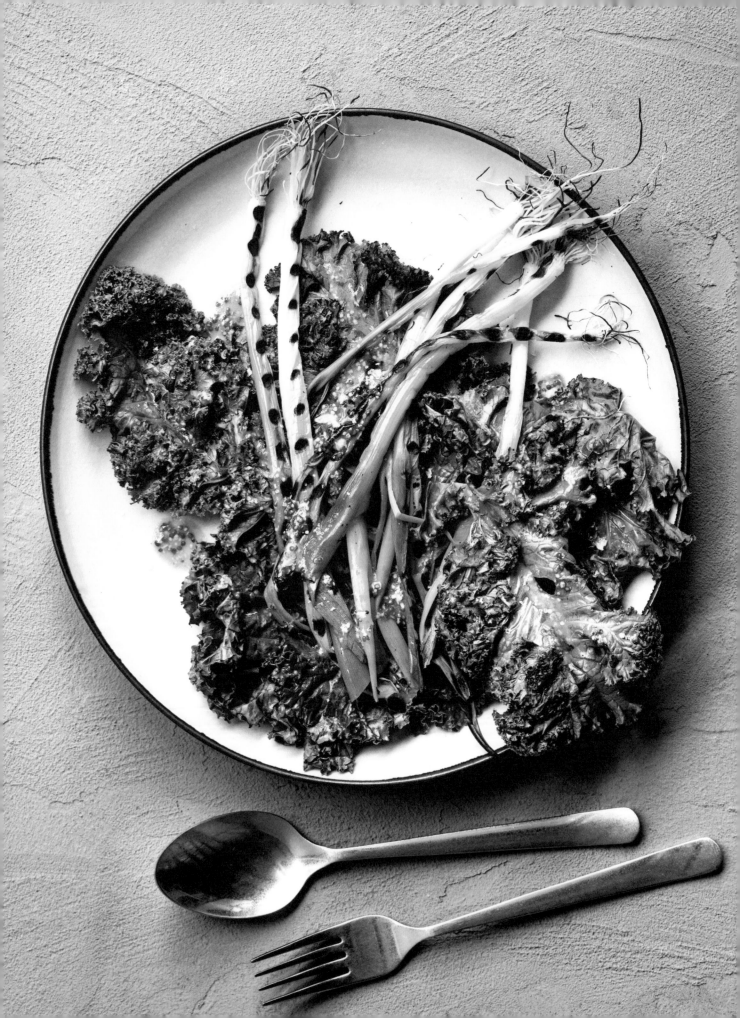

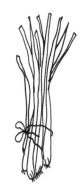

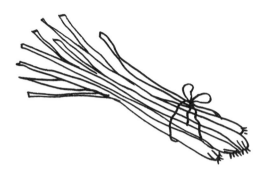

BARBECUED KALE *and* SPRING ONION *with* GARLIC

SERVES: 4 AS A SIDE

	PER SERVE
ENERGY (KJ/CAL)	281/67
PROTEIN (G)	2
FAT (G)	4.5
SATURATED FAT (G)	0.5
CARBOHYDRATE (G)	3.5

TOBIE I was lucky enough to cook with the uber-talented Darren Robertson on his TV show, *Charcoal Kitchen*, and he did a version of this dish. I went straight home and cooked it my own way and I love it. The spring onions become so delicious and sweet when grilled. This one's for you, Darren.

Preheat the barbecue and grill plate on high.

Place the garlic cloves and lemon half, flesh side down, on the hottest part of the barbecue. Cook the garlic until darkened underneath, then turn and cook the other side. Cook the lemon until the flesh is dark in colour, then remove and set aside. When the garlic is cooked, place it on a chopping board and leave to cool a little before peeling away the skin and placing the flesh in a small bowl.

Wash the kale thoroughly and put it on the hot barbecue – you want it to still be a little wet, as the water will become steam and speed up the cooking process. Cook the kale until it just starts to blacken around the edges, then turn and repeat for the other side. (You may need to cook the kale in batches, depending on the size of your barbecue.) Transfer to a large bowl.

Lastly, put the spring onions on the barbecue and cook until softened and the edges start to darken. Transfer to a plate.

Use a fork to mash the garlic, then squeeze in the juice and pulp of the grilled lemon. Add the olive oil and mustard and stir to combine.

Cut the kale into thick strips and put on a serving platter with the spring onion. Drizzle over the garlic and lemon dressing and use tongs to turn the vegetables to coat. Season with salt and pepper, and serve right away.

2 cloves garlic, unpeeled

½ lemon

1 bunch curly kale, stalks trimmed

1 bunch spring onions, tops trimmed

1 tablespoon extra virgin olive oil

1 teaspoon gluten-free wholegrain mustard

sea salt and cracked black pepper

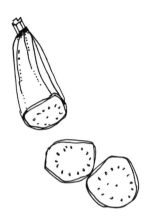

GRILLED ZUCCHINI *with* MINT, FETA *and* PINE NUTS

SERVES: 4 AS A SIDE

	PER SERVE
ENERGY (KJ/CAL)	616/147
PROTEIN (G)	5.5
FAT (G)	12
SATURATED FAT (G)	2
CARBOHYDRATE (G)	3.5

1½ tablespoons pine nuts

600 g zucchini (courgettes) (about 4–6), trimmed

1 lemon, halved

sea salt and cracked black pepper

handful of basil leaves

handful of mint leaves

1 tablespoon extra virgin olive oil

50 g reduced-fat goat's milk feta

TOBIE When I left the restaurant kitchen and started exploring cuisines other than my beloved Italian, I came home armed with some feta cheese and now I'm totally addicted to it. Zucchini and mint is a combo I've been making for years, but the touch of saltiness from a scattering of feta really lifts it to another level. This is the kind of dish that works with more or less anything and makes a delicious lunch teamed with a quinoa salad.

Preheat the barbecue grill on high.

Put the pine nuts in a dry frying pan over medium heat and toast until golden, about 2 minutes. Transfer to a small bowl.

Cut the zucchini diagonally into slices about 1 cm thick. Put on the hot grill in a single layer and cook for 2 minutes each side or until grill marks are visible. While the zucchini is cooking, add the lemon halves to the grill, flesh side down, and cook for 5 minutes or until the flesh is quite dark in colour.

When the zucchini is cooked, transfer to a large bowl, add the toasted pine nuts and sprinkle with a pinch of both salt and pepper. Tear in the herbs, then squeeze over the grilled lemon juice and drizzle with the olive oil. Use your hands to toss the ingredients together and serve with the feta crumbled over the top.

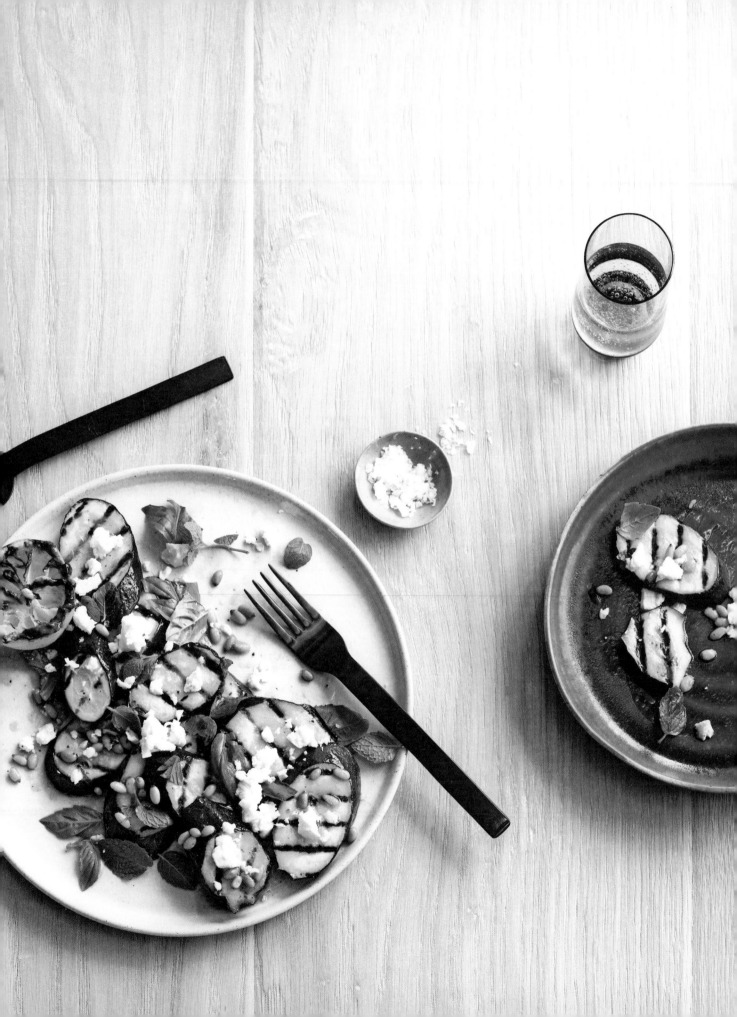

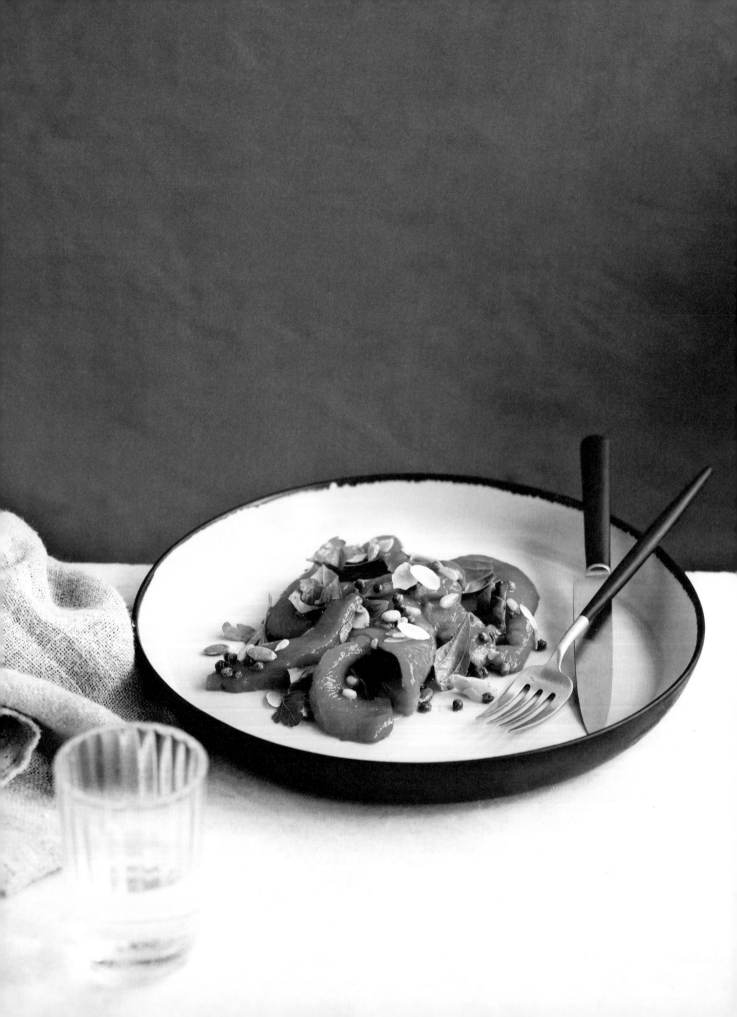

ROAST CAPSICUM *with* CAPERS, SEEDS *and* NUTS

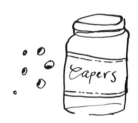

TOBIE One of my first jobs as an apprentice chef was to cook, peel and marinate copious amounts of capsicum. I had to make sure it was pretty well submerged in olive oil to preserve it, however we always used it up quickly so this seemed unnecessary to me. There's hardly any oil in this recipe as it's only used for flavour, and you can use almond or flaxseed oil if you like.

GEORGIA When capsicum is roasted it becomes really soft and sweet – it tastes quite different to raw capsicum. This makes a lovely side dish and if there's any left over (which doesn't happen often), I like to throw it into my salad for lunch the next day.

Preheat the oven to 200°C. Line a baking tray with baking paper.

Place the capsicums on the lined tray and bake for 20 minutes or until the skin is blistered and blackened all over. Remove from the oven and use tongs to immediately transfer to a large heatproof bowl – take care, they will be super-hot. Wrap the bowl very tightly with plastic film and then set aside for 15 minutes. (The steam from the capsicums will become trapped in the bowl and this helps to loosen the skins from the flesh.)

Use your fingers to remove and discard the skin, seeds and core of the capsicums. (Doing this under cold running water does make it easier, but I try to avoid this as one of my very respected ex-bosses, Rose Gray, told me we lose the flavour of the capsicum by doing so.) Tear the flesh into strips.

Place the capsicum strips in a large bowl and add the olive oil, vinegar and a good grind of pepper. Use tongs to gently toss the capsicum to coat in the dressing. Add the seed and nut mix, capers and herbs and carefully toss or fold to combine. Serve right away.

SERVES: 4 AS A SIDE

	PER SERVE
ENERGY (KJ/CAL)	519/124
PROTEIN (G)	3.5
FAT (G)	10
SATURATED FAT (G)	1.5
CARBOHYDRATE (G)	4

3 capsicums (peppers)

1 tablespoon extra virgin olive oil

2 teaspoons apple cider vinegar

cracked black pepper

2 tablespoons Seed and nut mix (see page 190)

2 tablespoons salted baby capers, rinsed

handful of flat-leaf parsley, roughly chopped

handful of basil leaves, roughly torn

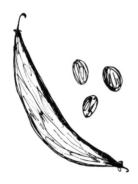

KALE *with* ROAST TOMATOES *and* BORLOTTI BEANS

SERVES: 4 AS A SIDE

	PER SERVE
ENERGY (KJ/CAL)	827/198
PROTEIN (G)	4
FAT (G)	15.5
SATURATED FAT (G)	2.5
CARBOHYDRATE (G)	9

250 g mixed small tomatoes (such as cherry, grape and teardrop)

¼ cup (60 ml) extra virgin olive oil

1 teaspoon thyme leaves, roughly chopped

sea salt and cracked black pepper

1 large bunch curly kale

2 cloves garlic, thinly sliced

1 red bird's-eye chilli, finely chopped (optional)

100 g rinsed and drained tinned borlotti beans

handful of black olives (such as kalamata), pitted

TOBIE This dish is as delicious eaten cold as it is warm, served as a side with any of the protein recipes from this book. You can cook your own borlotti beans, of course, but with so many great-quality tinned pulses available I often opt for them to save time.

Preheat the oven to 180°C. Line a baking tray with baking paper.

Toss the tomatoes, 1 tablespoon of olive oil, the thyme and a pinch of both salt and pepper together in a bowl. Spread the tomatoes over the lined tray and roast for 20 minutes or until the skins start to blister and darken.

Meanwhile, remove the stalks from the kale (I normally cut them off about 3 cm below the leaf). Thickly slice the leaves, then wash well in cold water. Transfer to a colander to dry a little.

Heat the remaining olive oil in a large heavy-based saucepan over low–medium heat. Add the garlic and chilli, if using, and cook gently for 2–3 minutes, until the garlic softens but isn't coloured. Increase the heat to medium–high and add the borlotti beans, olives and half of the roasted tomatoes. Cook, stirring, for 1 minute before adding the kale (the pan may look crowded at this stage, but the kale will soon wilt). Continue to stir the kale so that nothing sticks to the base of the pan. If the base of the pan is becoming dry, add a tablespoon of water – the steam that is created will also help the kale cook a little faster.

After 3–4 minutes the kale will be softened and vibrant green in colour. Remove the pan from the heat, gently stir through the remaining tomatoes and season with a good pinch of both salt and pepper. Serve right away.

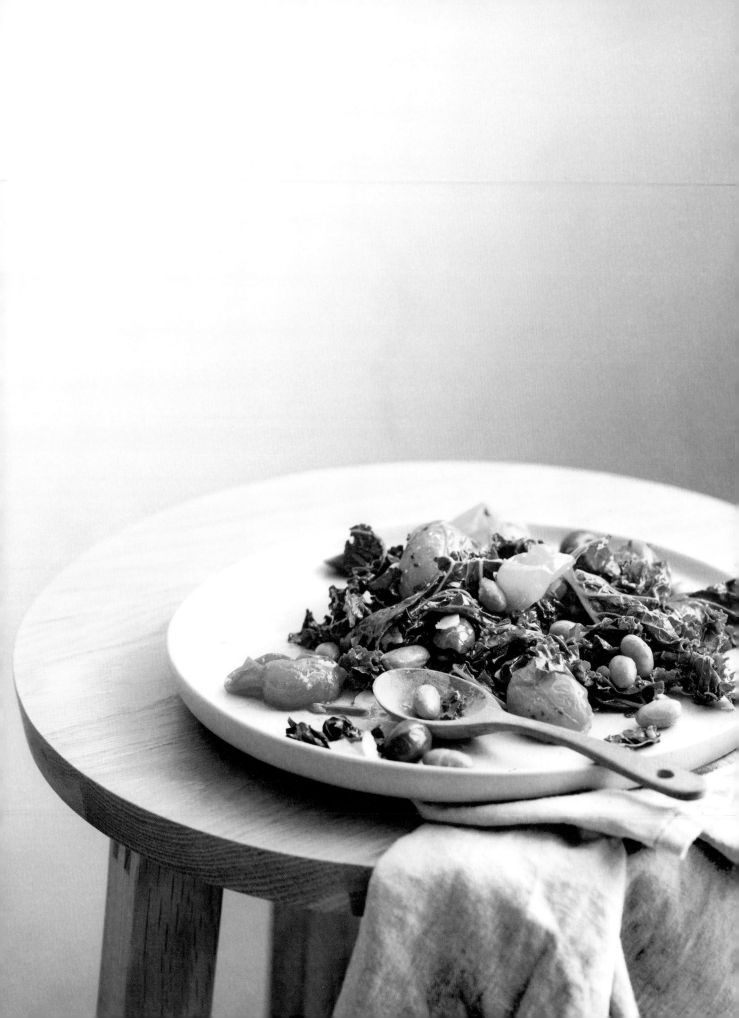

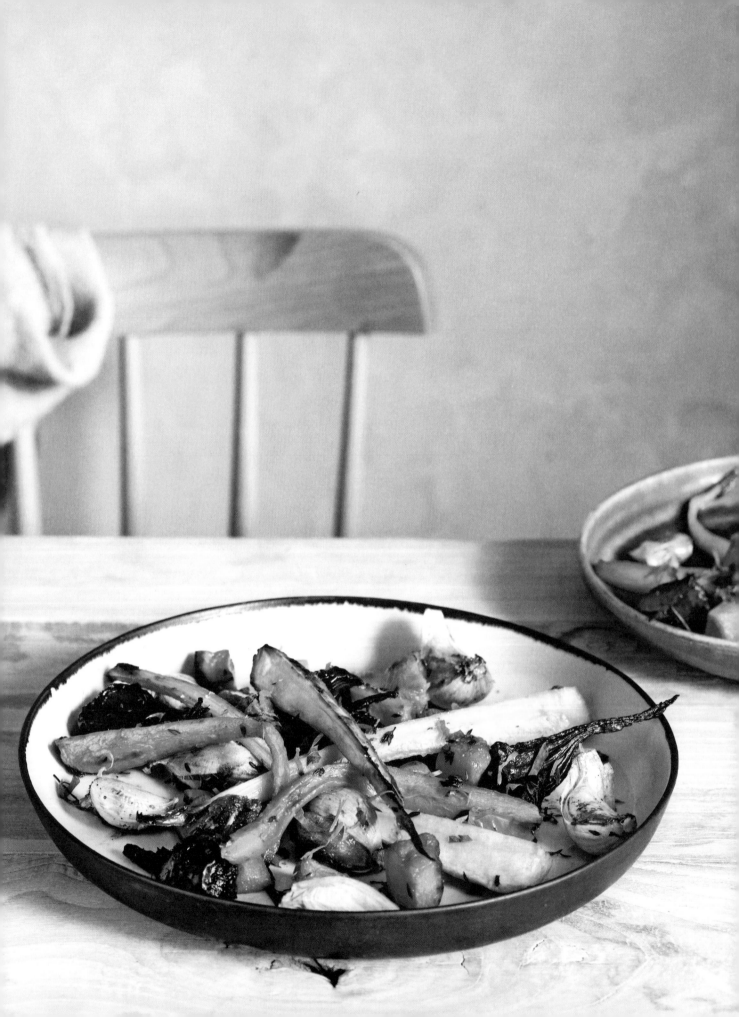

ROASTED ROOT VEGETABLES

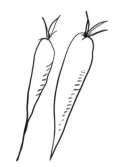

TOBIE Georgia *loves* a Sunday roast. But Georgia doesn't eat meat, potatoes are out and you can forget about using duck fat. So the compromise is this – simple, well-seasoned and perfectly cooked root vegetables that are great for dinner, beautiful eaten cold for lunch and make amazing bubble and squeak (see page 29).

Preheat the oven to 200°C. Line a large baking tray with baking paper.

Put all the vegetables in a large bowl and add the olive oil, honey, thyme and a good pinch of both salt and pepper.

Scatter the vegetables over the lined tray, spreading them out in a single layer so they cook evenly (use a second tray if necessary). Scatter the garlic cloves over the vegetables. Roast the vegetables for 40 minutes or until they are golden and tender.

Transfer the vegetables and garlic to a serving platter. Scatter over the parsley, season with salt and pepper and serve.

SERVES: 6 AS A SIDE

	PER SERVE
ENERGY (KJ/CAL)	834/200
PROTEIN (G)	4.5
FAT (G)	6.5
SATURATED FAT (G)	1
CARBOHYDRATE (G)	26

1 sweet potato (about 300 g), peeled and cut into 2 cm cubes

3 carrots (about 300 g in total), quartered lengthways

3 parsnips (about 300 g in total), peeled and quartered lengthways

300 g celeriac, peeled and cut into 2 cm cubes

1 bunch baby beetroots (about 300 g), trimmed and halved

2 tablespoons extra virgin olive oil

1 tablespoon honey

2 tablespoons thyme leaves

sea salt and cracked black pepper

12 cloves garlic, unpeeled

handful of flat-leaf parsley, roughly shredded

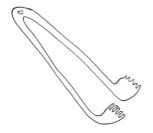

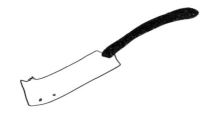

BARBECUED ASPARAGUS
and BROCCOLINI

SERVES: 4 AS A SIDE

	PER SERVE
ENERGY (KJ/CAL)	384/92
PROTEIN (G)	6
FAT (G)	5
SATURATED FAT (G)	0.5
CARBOHYDRATE (G)	2.5

1 tablespoon extra virgin olive oil

6 anchovy fillets (optional)

1 clove garlic, finely chopped

150 g cherry tomatoes

400 g asparagus, ends trimmed

2 bunches (350 g) broccolini, ends trimmed

sea salt and cracked black pepper

handful of basil leaves

TOBIE I love barbecuing greens because they taste so good, but there's an added bonus in that they also retain more nutrients than, say, boiling them. I used to toss the greens in extra virgin olive oil with a generous amount of seasoning before barbecuing, but I've found that putting them in a mixture of oil, garlic and anchovy fillets after cooking gives an exceptional flavour.

I have a small barbie at home and I always cook over coals. For this particular recipe I love nothing more than to hit the tomatoes with just a little smoke. If you have a coal barbecue and you'd like to try this, cook the tomatoes last and when they're nearly done add just a few woodchips to the coals (check the instructions on the packaging to see if the woodchips need to be soaked first), then cover the barbie and smoke the tomatoes for 5 minutes or so.

Preheat the barbecue or grill plate on high.

Put the oil, anchovies, if using, and garlic in a heatproof metal bowl just off-centre on the barbecue and let the oil heat up a little. Dip your finger in to test the temperature and when it is quite warm remove the bowl from the heat and use a fork to stir the anchovies into the oil, allowing them to break down. Place the bowl in a warm spot close to the barbecue.

Place the tomatoes on the barbecue and cook until they are just starting to blister and burst, then add them to the bowl with the oil mixture.

Place the asparagus and broccolini on the barbecue and flick a small amount of water over them while they cook, to help them steam through a little. When they start to darken underneath, turn and cook the other side. I generally cook mine for about 5 minutes all up. When they are ready, add them to the bowl with the tomatoes and use some tongs to carefully turn to coat in the oil mixture.

Have a taste and season with salt and pepper – remember if you're using anchovies they will add salt, too. Tear in the basil and serve right away.

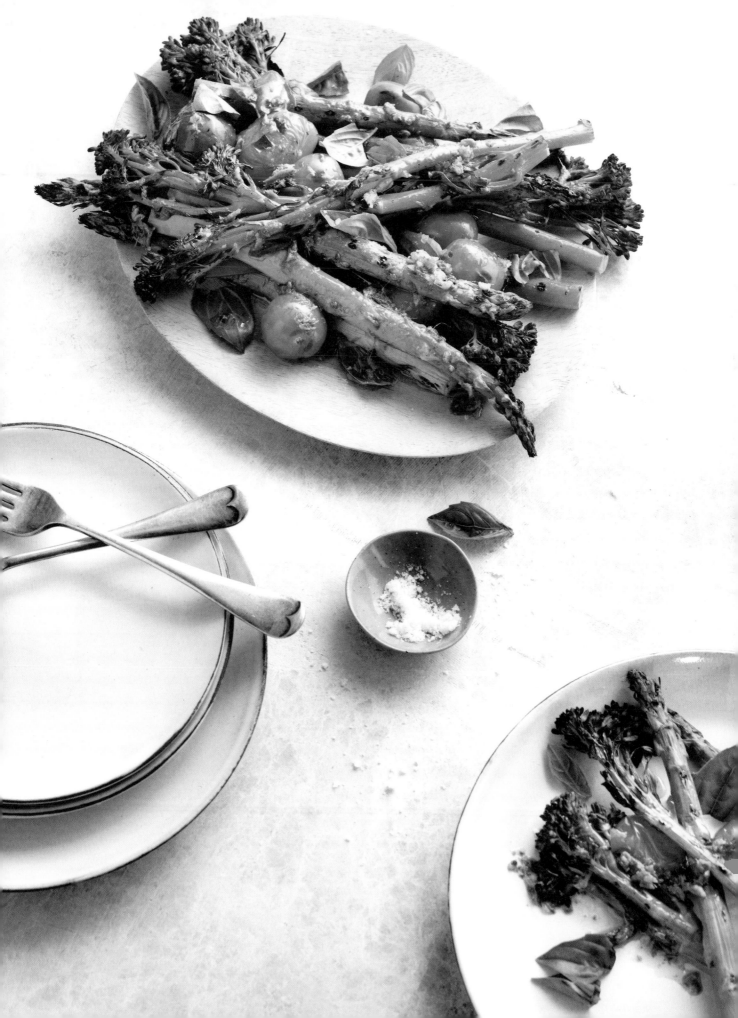

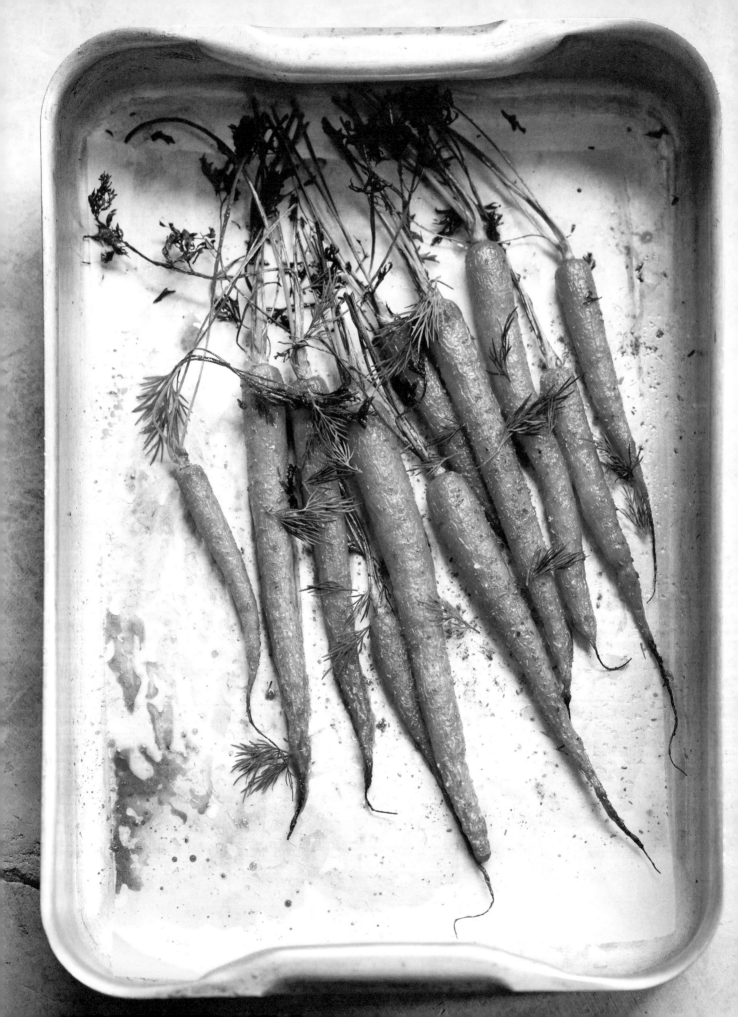

ROAST CARROTS with HONEY, CUMIN and DILL

TOBIE This dish is a great example of the way just one or two complementary flavours can really showcase the beauty of good seasonal produce. The honey helps caramelise the carrots as they roast, giving them a beautiful sweetness. You could also use regular carrots, just quarter them lengthways.

GEORGIA Good-quality ingredients make all the difference to simple dishes such as this. On that note, Manuka honey and Murray River or Maldon salt will really make it a winner.

600 g baby (Dutch) carrots, scrubbed

1 tablespoon extra virgin olive oil

1 tablespoon honey

1 heaped teaspoon ground cumin

sea salt and cracked black pepper

small handful of roughly chopped dill

Preheat the oven to 220°C. Line a roasting pan with baking paper.

Put the carrots, olive oil, honey, cumin, a large pinch of salt and some pepper in a bowl and toss until the carrots are well coated. Spread the carrots in a single layer over the lined pan and roast for 30–40 minutes or until caramelised and tender.

Sprinkle the carrots with the dill and serve.

SERVES: 4 AS A SIDE

	PER SERVE
ENERGY (KJ/CAL)	471/113
PROTEIN (G)	1.5
FAT (G)	5
SATURATED FAT (G)	0.5
CARBOHYDRATE (G)	13.5

PARSNIP PUREE

TOBIE For the last 20 years I have been following a similar formula for vegetable purees. I cook the veggies in milk or a combination of cream/milk and stock, along with flavourings such as garlic, bay leaf and various other herbs, then I finish the puree with butter and cheese. The result is not surprising – a super-rich and decadent puree that will surely make itself apparent if you eat it too often. This version, on the other hand, is super-lean but it's still super-tasty.

3 parsnips (about 700 g in total), trimmed and peeled

1 large clove garlic, peeled

1 bay leaf

sea salt and cracked black pepper

2 teaspoons black or white truffle oil

Roughly chop the parsnips into equal-sized pieces – I usually go for chunks about the size of my thumb. Place in a heavy-based saucepan and cover with plenty of water. Add the garlic, bay leaf and a large pinch of salt.

Bring the water to the boil over high heat, then reduce the heat and hold at a gentle simmer for 30 minutes or until the parsnip is tender. Drain the parsnip, reserving 1 cup of the cooking water and discarding the bay leaf, and put in a food processor. Process to a smooth puree, adding some of the cooking water if needed to get the right consistency. Add the truffle oil, another pinch of salt and some pepper, to taste, and serve.

SERVES: 4 AS A SIDE

	PER SERVE
ENERGY (KJ/CAL)	480/115
PROTEIN (G)	3
FAT (G)	2.5
SATURATED FAT (G)	0.5
CARBOHYDRATE (G)	16.5

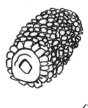

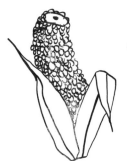

BARBECUED CORN
in the HUSK

SERVES: 4 AS A SIDE

	PER SERVE
ENERGY (KJ/CAL)	760/182
PROTEIN (G)	7
FAT (G)	8.5
SATURATED FAT (G)	2
CARBOHYDRATE (G)	15.5

4 corn cobs, husks intact

2 limes, halved

¼ cup (20 g) freshly grated asiago cheese (or parmesan)

handful of flat-leaf parsley or coriander, roughly chopped

1 teaspoon hot paprika

1 red bird's-eye chilli, finely chopped (optional)

sea salt and cracked black pepper

1 tablespoon extra virgin olive oil

TOBIE I'm a big fan of corn, especially the Mexican-style barbecued corn with cheese and lime. In this version, I've used a little olive oil instead of butter and cut down on the cheese, so all that fabulous flavour is still there, without too much saturated fat.

GEORGIA Back in the day, I would have eaten my corn slathered in butter, but this delicious recipe proves you really don't need it.

Preheat the barbecue on high.

Place the corn cobs (still in the husks) on the hot barbecue and cook until the husks are blackened. Carefully peel away the blackened layer of husk from each cob and discard. Continue cooking, peeling away each layer of husk as it blackens until the entire husk has blackened and been removed. Continue to cook the corn cobs until the kernels start to colour just a little. This should take about 30 minutes all up. While the corn is cooking, add the lime halves to the barbecue, flesh side down, and cook for 5 minutes or until the flesh is dark in colour.

While the corn and lime are cooking, put the asiago, parsley or coriander, paprika, chilli, if using, and a good pinch of both salt and pepper in a bowl and use your fingers to mix well.

Remove the lime and corn from the barbecue. Rub the olive oil over the corn cobs to coat each, then quickly pop them into the bowl with the cheese, one at a time, and give a good shake to get as much of the cheese to stick to the corn cobs as possible.

Serve right away with the grilled lime wedges and sprinkled with any cheesy and chilli bits remaining in the bowl.

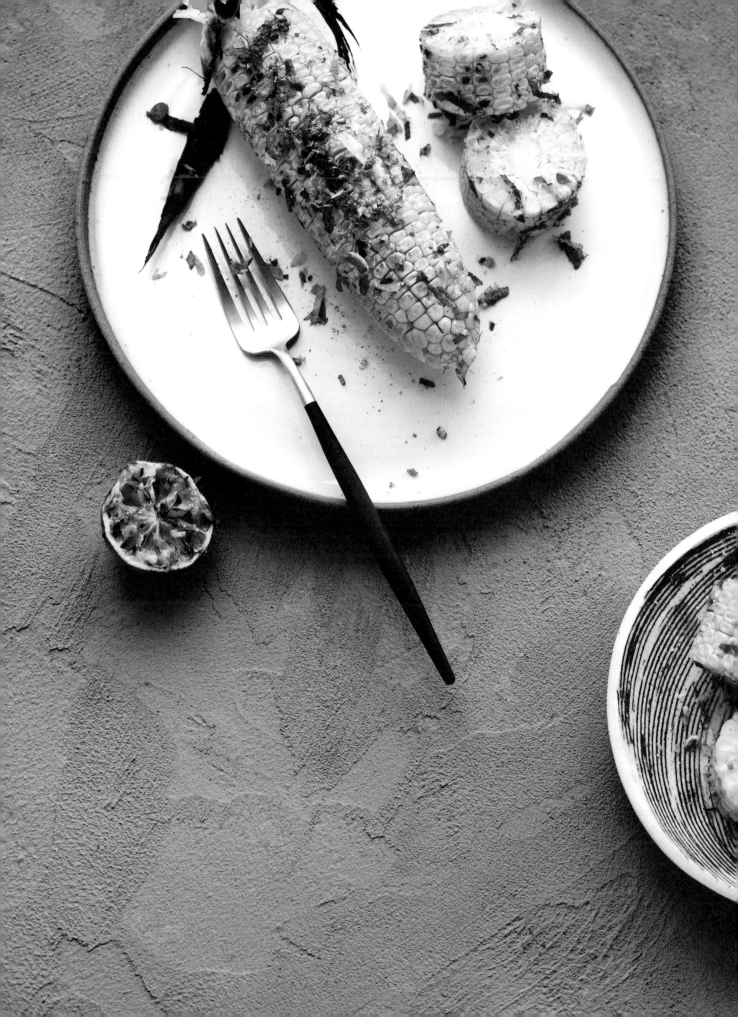

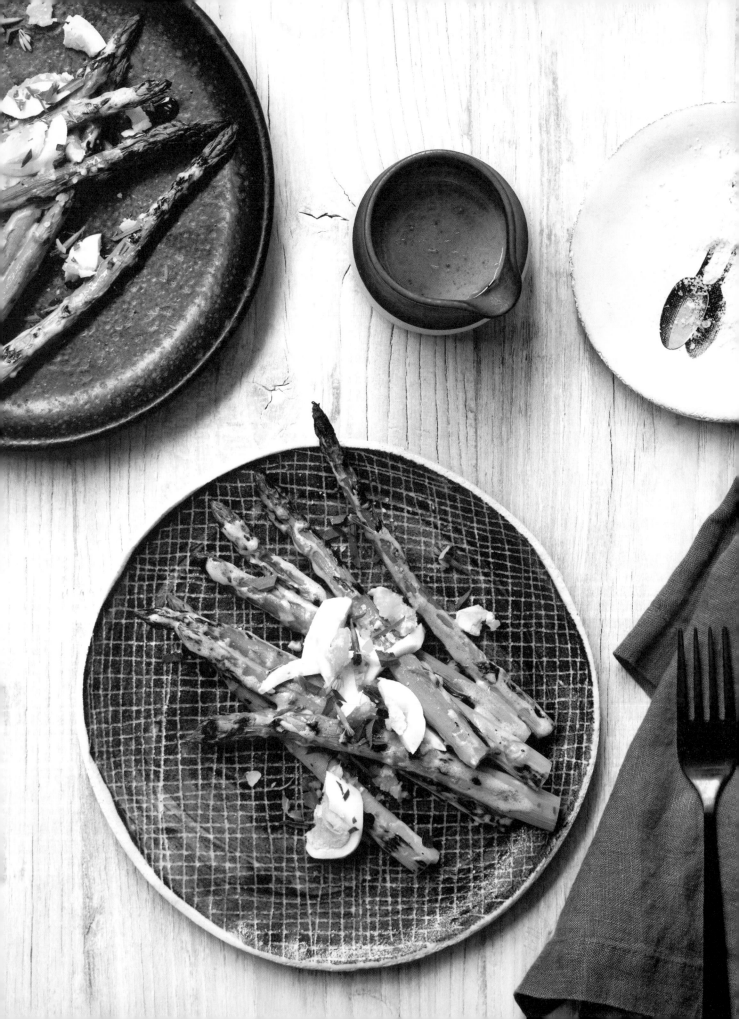

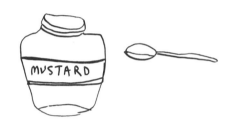

GRILLED ASPARAGUS *with* SOFT-BOILED EGGS, MUSTARD *and* TARRAGON

SERVES: 4 AS A SIDE OR
2 FOR LUNCH

	PER SERVE (FOR 4)
ENERGY (KJ/CAL)	390/93
PROTEIN (G)	5.5
FAT (G)	7
SATURATED FAT (G)	1.5
CARBOHYDRATE (G)	1.5

TOBIE Eggs, Dijon mustard and tarragon are amazing together, and when you combine them with smoky charred asparagus you'll wonder why you ever ordered takeaway.

Put the eggs in a small saucepan and cover with cold water. Bring the water to a gentle simmer, then remove from the heat, cover with the lid and set aside for 15 minutes. Transfer the eggs to a colander or sieve and sit under cold running water until cooled. Peel the eggs and set aside until needed.

Preheat a grill plate or barbecue on high. Put the asparagus on the hot grill or barbecue (there's no need to oil it first) and cook for 10–15 minutes or until tender, turning the spears from time to time so they cook evenly.

While the asparagus is cooking, combine the mustard, olive oil and red wine vinegar in a large bowl.

Add the asparagus to the dressing and use tongs to turn the spears to coat evenly. Place on serving plates or a large platter. Roughly chop the eggs and scatter over the asparagus, along with the tarragon. Season with a good pinch of both salt and pepper and serve right away.

2 eggs

20 asparagus spears (about 260 g in total), ends trimmed

2 teaspoons gluten-free Dijon mustard

1 tablespoon extra virgin olive oil

2 teaspoons red wine vinegar

small handful of tarragon leaves, roughly chopped

sea salt and cracked black pepper

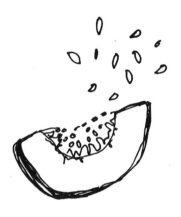

ROAST PUMPKIN *with* SEED *and* NUT TOPPING

SERVES: 4–6 AS A SIDE

	PER SERVE (FOR 6)
ENERGY (KJ/CAL)	950/227
PROTEIN (G)	7
FAT (G)	16
SATURATED FAT (G)	2
CARBOHYDRATE (G)	12

1½ tablespoons extra virgin olive oil

1 kg pumpkin (squash)

sea salt and cracked black pepper

1 cup (120 g) Seed and nut mix
(see page 190)

handful of flat-leaf parsley,
finely chopped

1 tablespoon finely chopped
marjoram leaves

1 red bird's-eye chilli, finely chopped

2 tablespoons finely grated
parmesan

TOBIE This dish is a hero in its own right, but it will go well as a side for most of the meat and fish dishes in this book. You can use kent (jap) or butternut pumpkin here.

GEORGIA Another ridiculously yummy dish, and again leftovers are great to add to lunch salads. The pumpkin becomes super-sweet when roasted and the nuts and seeds impart a beautiful texture.

Preheat the oven to 200°C. Line a baking tray with baking paper and drizzle 2 teaspoons of olive oil over the paper.

Use a large sharp knife to cut the pumpkin into wedges, about 1 cm thick, and remove the seeds. Place in a single layer on the prepared tray, then drizzle with 2 teaspoons of the remaining olive oil. Season with salt and pepper and bake for 15 minutes.

Meanwhile, put the seed and nut mix, parsley, marjoram, chilli, parmesan, remaining 2 teaspoons of olive oil and a good pinch of both salt and pepper in a bowl. Stir until well combined.

Remove the pumpkin from the oven. Turn all the wedges over, then scatter the seed and nut mixture over the top. Return to the oven for a further 15–20 minutes or until the pumpkin is tender. Serve.

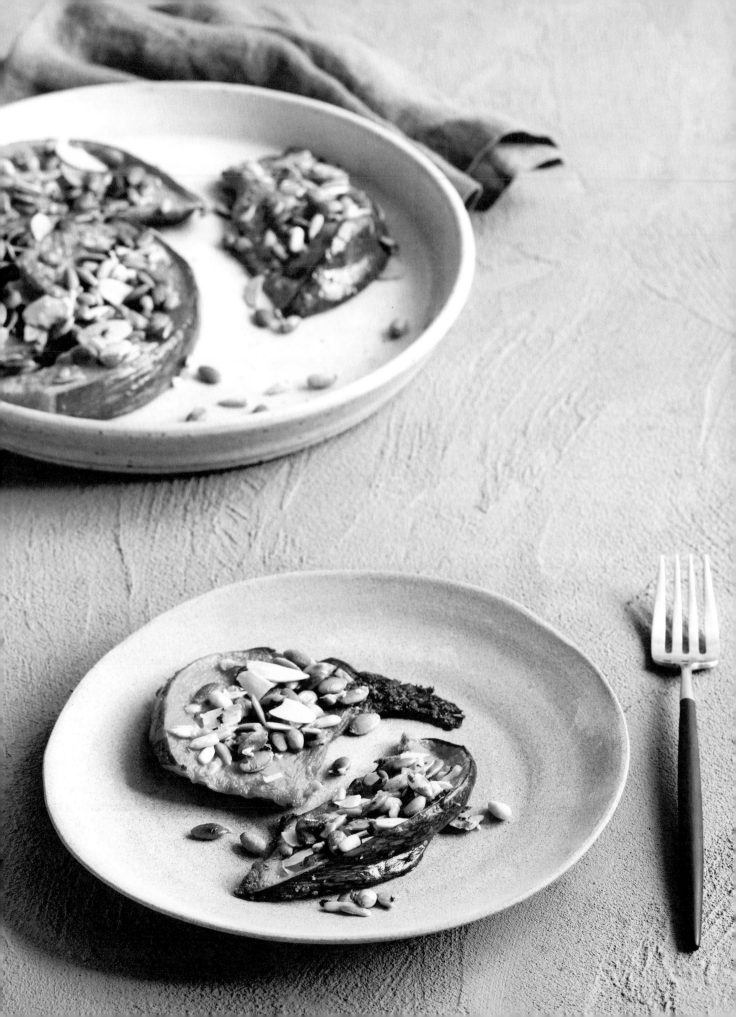

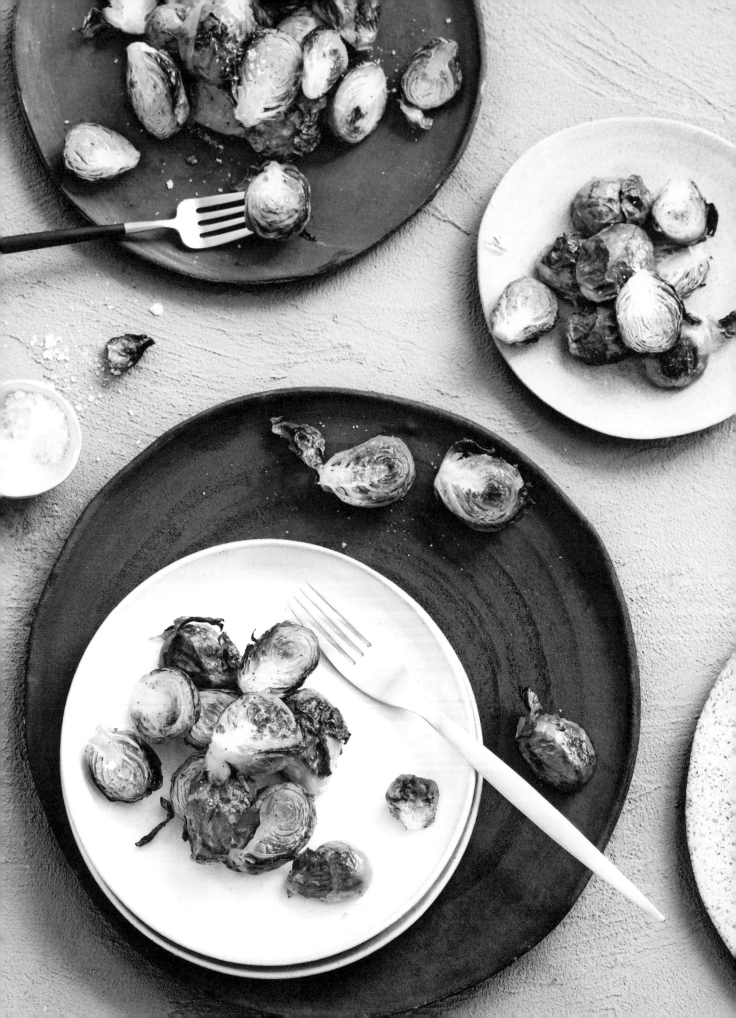

ROASTED BRUSSELS SPROUTS

TOBIE I've made these for friends and everyone thinks they're amazing, but the funny thing is that they are ridiculously simple to make. Extra virgin olive oil, salt and pepper, that's it. I think the trick to getting them nice and crisp is not to move them around too much while they are cooking. And when you think they are done, cook them for 5 minutes more.

500 g brussels sprouts

2 tablespoons extra virgin olive oil

good pinch of sea salt

good pinch of cayenne pepper

1 teaspoon dried chilli flakes (optional)

handful of flat-leaf parsley, finely chopped

Preheat the oven to 180°C. Line a baking tray with baking paper.

Trim the cores of the brussels sprouts, discard any tough outer leaves and then cut each one in half. Place in a large bowl, add the olive oil, salt, cayenne pepper and chilli, if using, and toss to combine.

Spread the brussels sprouts over the lined tray in a single layer and roast for 15–20 minutes or until tender and browned. Return the brussels sprouts to the bowl, toss through the parsley and serve.

SERVES: 4 AS A SIDE

	PER SERVE
ENERGY (KJ/CAL)	534/128
PROTEIN (G)	5
FAT (G)	9.5
SATURATED FAT (G)	1.5
CARBOHYDRATE (G)	3

SWEET POTATO MASH

TOBIE This is a great dish to make each week and keep in the fridge for whenever you need a little something on the side. It heats up pretty nicely in the microwave, too.

1 kg sweet potatoes, peeled and cut into 3 cm pieces

2 bay leaves

2 tablespoons extra virgin olive oil

2 cloves garlic, finely chopped

1 red bird's-eye chilli, finely chopped

½ teaspoon freshly grated nutmeg

sea salt and cracked black pepper

Pop the sweet potato and bay leaves in a heavy-based saucepan, cover with cold water and bring to the boil over high heat. Reduce the heat and hold at a simmer for 30 minutes or until the sweet potato is tender.

While the sweet potato is cooking, put the olive oil, garlic and chilli in a small saucepan over low heat and cook for 2–3 minutes, until the garlic is softened. (The idea is to infuse the oil with the garlic and chilli without heating it up too much.)

Drain the sweet potato and discard the bay leaves, then transfer to a large bowl and use a potato masher to mash. Add the oil mixture, nutmeg and a good pinch of both salt and pepper and mix well. Taste and adjust the seasoning, if needed, and serve.

SERVES: 6 AS A SIDE

	PER SERVE
ENERGY (KJ/CAL)	826/198
PROTEIN (G)	4
FAT (G)	6.5
SATURATED FAT (G)	1
CARBOHYDRATE (G)	29

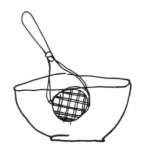

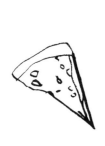
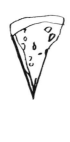

CAULIFLOWER PIZZA *with* EGGPLANT *and* MOZZARELLA

SERVES: 2

	PER SERVE
ENERGY (KJ/CAL)	1493/357
PROTEIN (G)	30.5
FAT (G)	18
SATURATED FAT (G)	7
CARBOHYDRATE (G)	11.5

600 g cauliflower florets

1 egg

1 tablespoon finely grated parmesan

sea salt and cracked black pepper

1 eggplant (aubergine)

½ quantity Napoli sauce (see page 187)

100 g low-fat mozzarella (or fior di latte if you want to be cheeky)

5 anchovy fillets

basil leaves, to serve

TOBIE This recipe was a real revelation; it's amazing how the cauliflower turns into a perfectly crisp crust. Remember whenever you make pizza not to overload it with toppings – do as the Italians do and practise a little 'less is more'. It tastes better and makes for a healthier meal.

GEORGIA We used to have pizza every Monday night. It was a ritual. A whole pizza each and a big glass of red wine or beer. We LOVE pizza, especially the delicious thin-based ones from our local pizzerias. Giving that up was really hard, but it had no place in our nutritious eating plan. Tobie played around with this recipe and I think it's perfect. You can pick up the slices just like real pizza, and I no longer feel like I'm missing out. This is my favourite topping, but you can put whatever you like on it.

Roughly chop the cauliflower florets and core and put in a food processor. Pulse until very finely chopped.

Bring a saucepan of salted water to the boil over high heat. Add the cauliflower and cook for 5 minutes, then drain in a fine-meshed sieve and refresh under cold running water. Tip the cauliflower onto a clean tea towel and wring out any excess moisture.

Transfer the cauliflower to a bowl and add the egg, parmesan and a little pinch of both salt and pepper. Mix well, then wrap in plastic film and place in the fridge for at least 30 minutes (or up to 24 hours).

While the dough is chilling, preheat the oven to 230°C. Line a 27.5 cm pizza tray with baking paper.

Preheat the barbecue or grill plate on medium–high. Cut the eggplant lengthways into 5 mm thick slices, place on the hot barbecue or grill and cook for 3–5 minutes each side or until grill marks are visible and the eggplant is soft and pliable. Set aside.

Remove the cauliflower dough from the fridge and use your fingers to press it over the lined tray so it covers the base evenly. It should be flat and firmly pressed onto the tray. Bake for 20–25 minutes or until browned and firm to the touch.

Remove the pizza base from the oven. Spread evenly with the Napoli sauce, then tear over the grilled eggplant and mozzarella. Lay the anchovies on top. Bake for 5–6 minutes or until the cheese is melted and starting to bubble. Remove from the oven, scatter over the basil and serve right away.

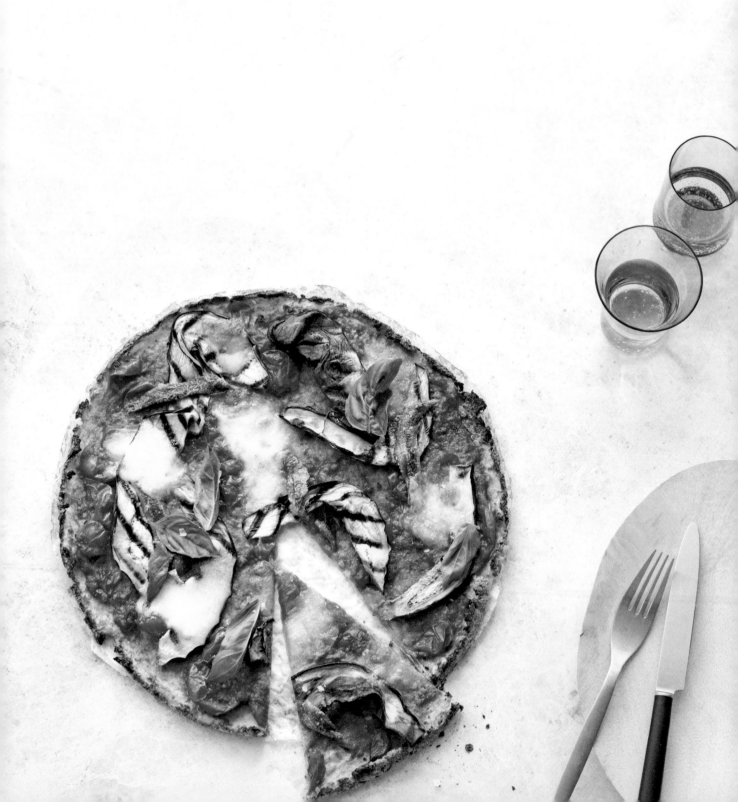

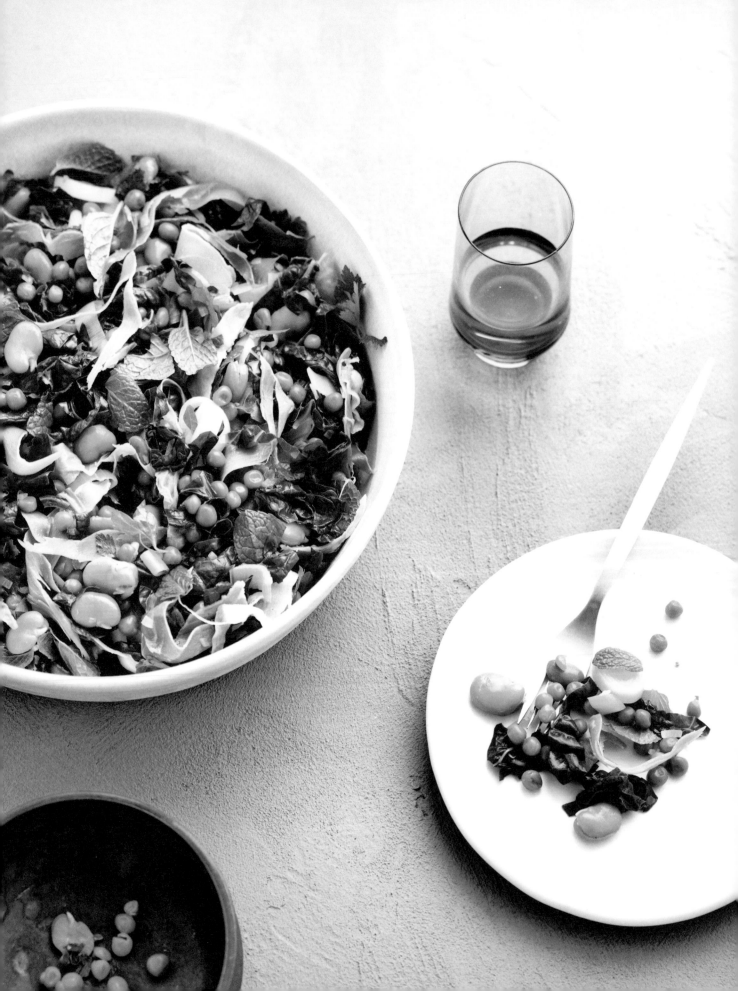

STEWED SPRING VEGETABLES

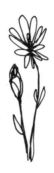

SERVES: 4 AS A SIDE

	PER SERVE
ENERGY (KJ/CAL)	680/163
PROTEIN (G)	10.5
FAT (G)	6
SATURATED FAT (G)	1.5
CARBOHYDRATE (G)	14

TOBIE I got the idea for this recipe from a dish I cooked at The River Café in London called *vignole*. It's often prepared with artichokes, peas, broad beans and other spring vegetables. In this version I use readily available ingredients and I've also reduced the cooking time a little to hang onto as many of the nutrients as possible. The prosciutto brings a delicious saltiness and depth of flavour, but if you don't eat meat it's still amazing without it.

Bring a large saucepan of salted water to the boil over high heat. Add the broad beans and blanch for around 1 minute, then use a slotted spoon to transfer to a bowl. Add the leek to the pan and blanch for 3 minutes or until tender, then use a slotted spoon to transfer to the bowl with the broad beans. Finally, blanch the silverbeet leaves for 1 minute, until wilted, then use a slotted spoon to transfer to the bowl with the other vegetables.

Heat the olive oil in a large heavy-based saucepan over medium heat. Add the shallot and cook gently, stirring often, until soft and translucent. Add the stock or water and bring to a gentle simmer. Add the peas, then scatter over the prosciutto, if using, and cook for 2 minutes or until the peas are nice and soft. Stir in the broad beans, leek and silverbeet and simmer for 2 minutes.

Season with salt and pepper, stir through the parsley and mint and leave to rest for 2 minutes before serving.

350 g double-podded broad beans

1 leek, white part only, washed well and thinly sliced into rounds

200 g silverbeet (Swiss chard), stalks removed, leaves washed and roughly sliced

1 tablespoon extra virgin olive oil

2 golden shallots, finely diced

300 ml gluten-free chicken or vegetable stock, or water

350 g shelled fresh peas (or frozen peas)

5–6 slices prosciutto, thinly sliced (optional)

sea salt and cracked black pepper

2 small handfuls of flat-leaf parsley leaves

2 small handfuls of mint leaves

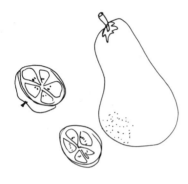

ROAST EGGPLANT with TOMATO, CAPERS and BASIL

SERVES: 4 AS A SIDE

	PER SERVE
ENERGY (KJ/CAL)	366/88
PROTEIN (G)	4
FAT (G)	3.5
SATURATED FAT (G)	0.5
CARBOHYDRATE (G)	7

2 large eggplants (aubergines), trimmed and cut into 2 cm cubes

sea salt and cracked black pepper

2 teaspoons extra virgin olive oil

450 g mixed tomatoes (I use a variety of heirloom tomatoes)

4 anchovy fillets

2 cloves garlic, chopped

small handful of salted baby capers, rinsed

handful of basil leaves, roughly torn

TOBIE This is another dish I have taken from my Italian training and twisted to fit the requirements of this book, and it tastes awesome. The eggplant is traditionally fried, but I bake it in this healthier version and I think it actually tastes better this way.

GEORGIA These flavours were meant for each other. The eggplant soaks them up and delivers perfection with each mouthful.

Put the eggplant in a colander set over a bowl, sprinkle with a pinch of salt and let it sit for about an hour, then rinse under cold water and pat dry using paper towel.

Preheat the oven to 180°C. Line 2 baking trays with baking paper.

Spread the eggplant over a lined tray in a single layer, then season with a pinch of both salt and pepper and drizzle over the olive oil. Bake the eggplant for 30 minutes or until browned.

Meanwhile, pop the tomatoes, anchovies, garlic and a pinch of both salt and pepper in a large bowl and toss to combine. Scatter the tomato mixture over the other lined tray and bake for 15 minutes or until the tomatoes start to blister.

Transfer the tomato mixture to a large heavy-based saucepan over low heat, add the capers and gently fold in the eggplant. Warm through for 4–5 minutes to allow the flavours to combine. Taste and adjust the seasoning if necessary, fold through the basil and serve.

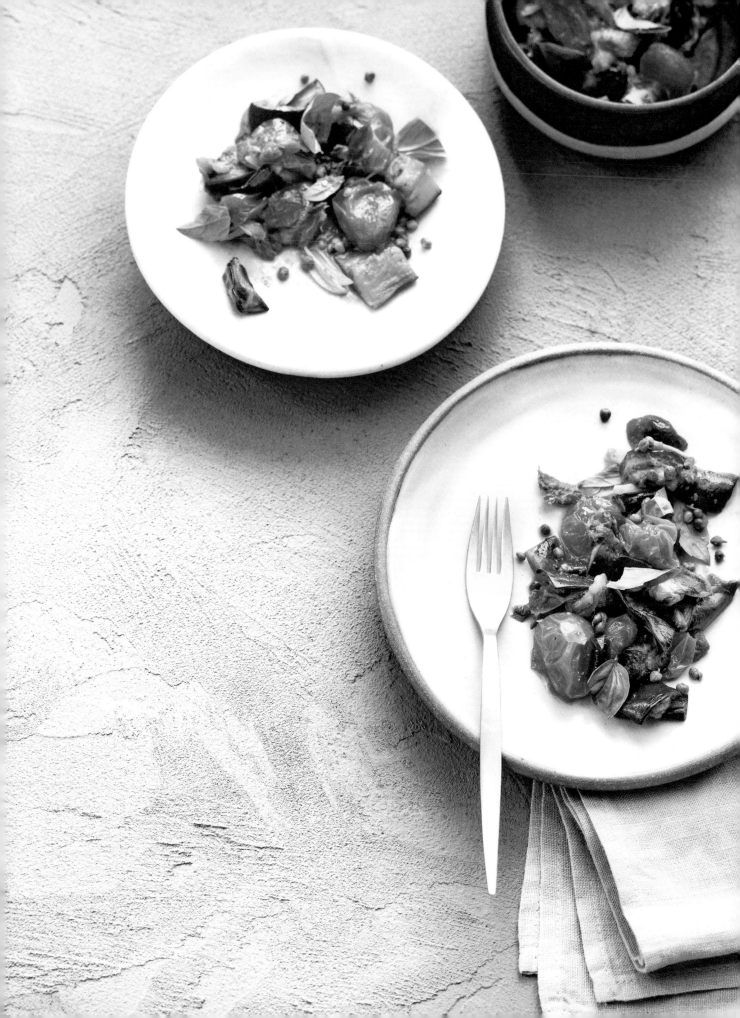

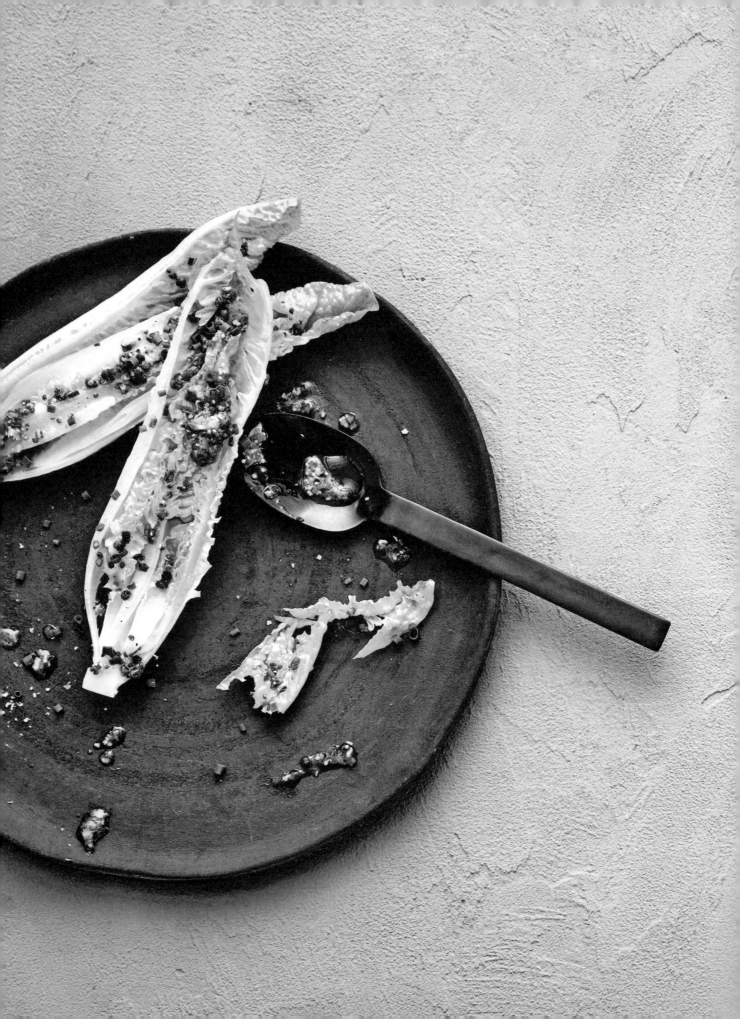

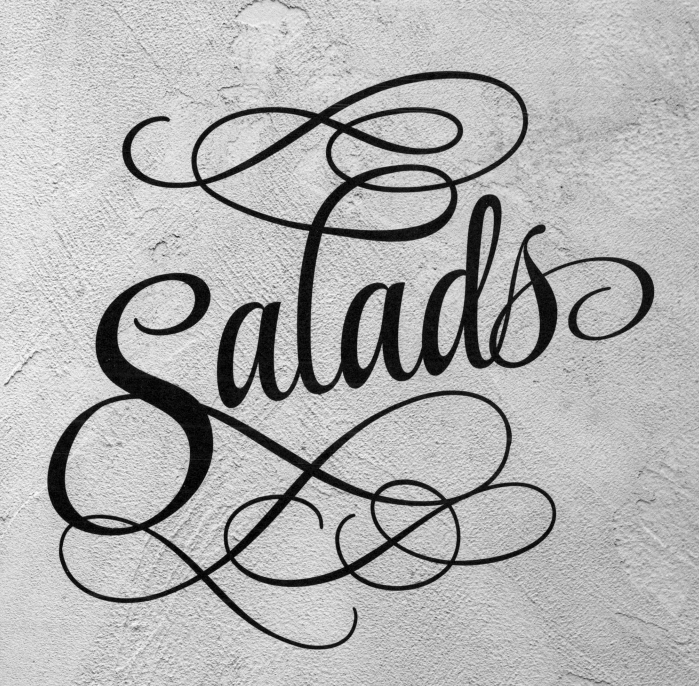

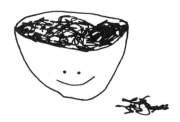

VERY NICE COLESLAW

SERVES: 6 AS A SIDE

	PER SERVE
ENERGY (KJ/CAL)	177/42
PROTEIN (G)	1.5
FAT (G)	2
SATURATED FAT (G)	0
CARBOHYDRATE (G)	3

¼ white cabbage, finely shredded

1 head radicchio, leaves separated and finely shredded

1 bulb fennel, trimmed and finely shredded

4 radishes, ends trimmed and finely shredded

handful of basil leaves, roughly torn

handful of mint leaves, roughly torn

handful of flat-leaf parsley leaves

1 tablespoon salted baby capers, rinsed

2 tablespoons Split anchovy and grilled lemon dressing (see page 189)

cracked black pepper

TOBIE I'm not really sure why I've called this coleslaw, because coleslaw doesn't usually have radicchio or fennel in it. But it does have shredded cabbage, so 'coleslaw' it is. This is hugely flexible and keeps well for about 24 hours, so when I make this recipe there are usually leftovers in Georgia's lunchbox the next day.

GEORGIA I used to think of coleslaw as a mayonnaisey, goopy mess. It wasn't something I ever went for, but this is fresh and yummy, and a perfect accompaniment for most types of protein.

Place the cabbage, radicchio, fennel, radish, basil, mint, parsley and capers in a large bowl. Drizzle over the dressing and season with pepper, then use your hands to gently toss the ingredients together. Serve right away.

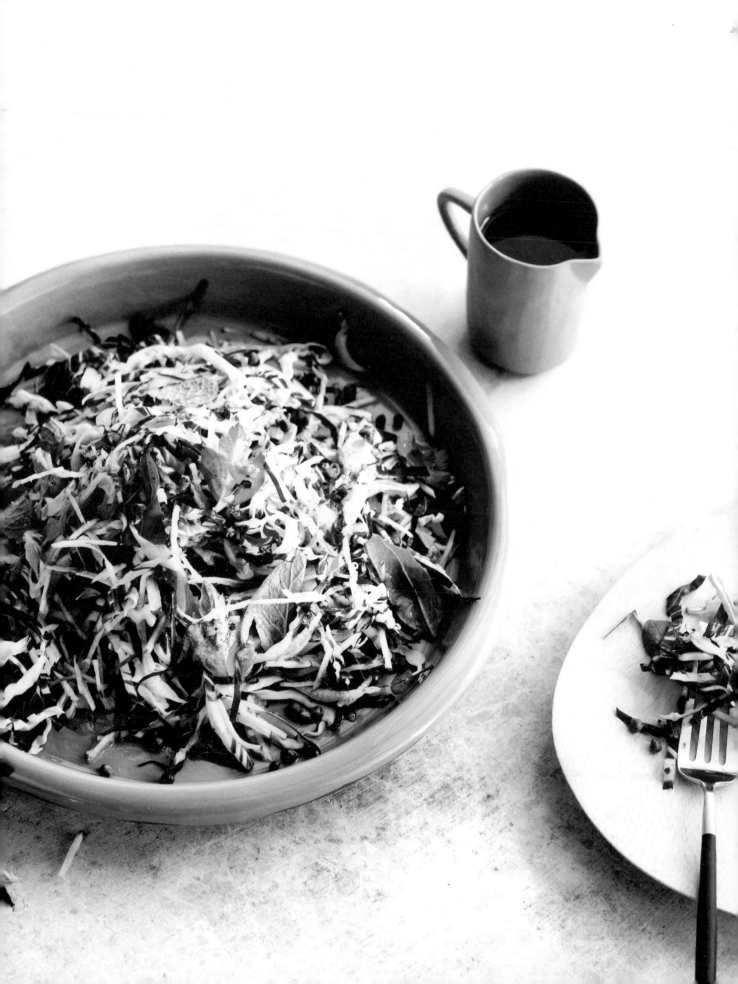

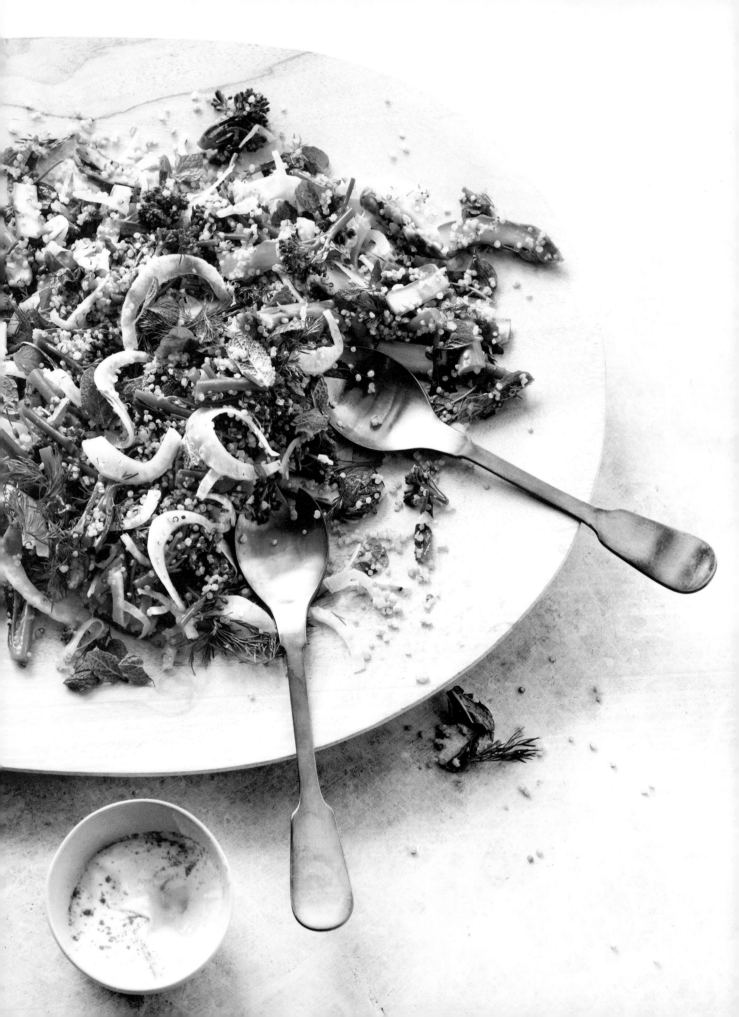

QUINOA, BROCCOLINI and ASPARAGUS SALAD

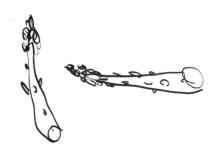

SERVES: 4 AS A SIDE

	PER SERVE
ENERGY (KJ/CAL)	909/217
PROTEIN (G)	9.5
FAT (G)	5
SATURATED FAT (G)	1
CARBOHYDRATE (G)	29.5

TOBIE When we first started writing this book we had a sort of section mapped out for take-to-work lunches, but when the book began to come together we realised that all the salad and vegetable recipes could work in this category. This is a case in point – it would be amazing with the roasted snapper on page 83 or eaten for lunch with some flaked smoked trout over the top.

Place the yoghurt in a bowl and season with salt and pepper. Finely chop half the mint leaves and mix into the yoghurt. Sprinkle with a pinch of cumin, then cover with plastic film and place in the fridge until needed.

Toast the quinoa in a heavy-based saucepan over medium heat, stirring constantly, for 2 minutes. Add 2 cups (500 ml) water and bring to the boil, then reduce the heat and hold at a simmer for 15 minutes. Turn off the heat and set aside, covered, for 5 minutes to allow the quinoa to absorb any remaining liquid. Transfer the quinoa to a large bowl and place in the fridge, uncovered, for about 10 minutes to cool.

Meanwhile, bring a saucepan of salted water to the boil and blanch the broccolini and asparagus for 1 minute, then drain and refresh under cold water to stop the cooking process. Set aside until needed.

Use a sharp knife to remove the stalks from the fennel bulb. Reserve the fronds and discard the stalks. Cut the fennel in half lengthways, then slice into thin strips and place in a bowl of iced water to keep it fresh and crisp. (You could also use a mandoline, or a vegetable peeler to peel long strips.)

Remove the cooled quinoa from the fridge. Add the broccolini, asparagus, fennel, capers, dill, lemon zest and juice, remaining mint leaves and pinch of cumin, reserved fennel fronds and a good drizzle of olive oil. Mix carefully so you don't bruise the herbs and then season with salt and pepper, to taste. Serve the quinoa salad with a dollop of the mint and cumin yoghurt on top.

2 heaped tablespoons low-fat plain Greek-style yoghurt

sea salt and cracked black pepper

2 small handfuls of mint leaves

2 pinches of ground cumin

¾ cup (150 g) quinoa

1 bunch broccolini, ends trimmed and cut into 3 cm lengths

1 bunch asparagus, ends trimmed and cut into 3 cm lengths

1 bulb baby fennel

1 tablespoon salted baby capers, rinsed and roughly chopped

1 small handful of dill, chopped

finely grated zest and juice of 1 lemon

extra virgin olive oil, for drizzling

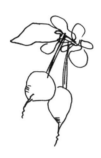

BEAN, RADISH and HAZELNUT SALAD with ANCHOVY and LEMON DRESSING

SERVES: 4 AS A SIDE

	PER SERVE
ENERGY (KJ/CAL)	793/190
PROTEIN (G)	5.5
FAT (G)	15.5
SATURATED FAT (G)	1
CARBOHYDRATE (G)	4.5

sea salt and cracked black pepper

300 g green beans, trimmed

200 g radishes, tops trimmed

80 g roasted and skinned hazelnuts, coarsely crushed

2 tablespoons Split anchovy and grilled lemon dressing (see page 189)

handful of mint leaves, roughly torn

TOBIE This combination was inspired by a lovely dish I had at a friend's house once. Their version had a caper and anchovy mayonnaise that was delicious but not particularly healthy, so I've replaced it with the anchovy and grilled lemon dressing from the pantry chapter. If you do not like anchovy, you can simply leave them out when making the dressing recipe.

GEORGIA I used to hate anchovies when I was a kid, but now I'm obsessed with them, especially the top-quality ones like the Ortiz brand. They are pure salty goodness and add so much flavour to a dish. This salad goes beautifully with a drained tin of tuna in springwater for lunch the next day.

Bring a saucepan of water to the boil and add a good pinch of salt. Add the beans and blanch for 2 minutes or until bright green and tender crisp, then drain and refresh in cold water to stop the cooking process. Set aside.

Rinse the radishes under cold water, then slice crossways as thinly as you can using a knife, mandoline or vegetable peeler. Place in a large bowl with the beans, hazelnuts and dressing. Using tongs, your hands or salad servers, toss the ingredients until they're evenly coated in the dressing. Add the mint and a good pinch of cracked black pepper, toss once again and serve.

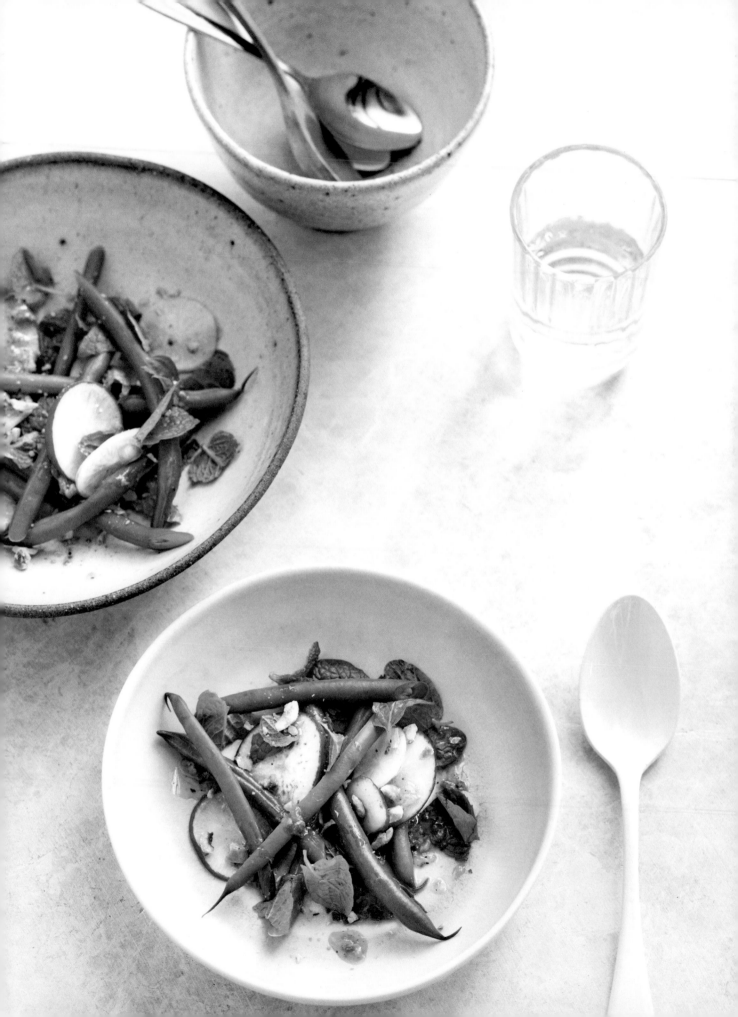

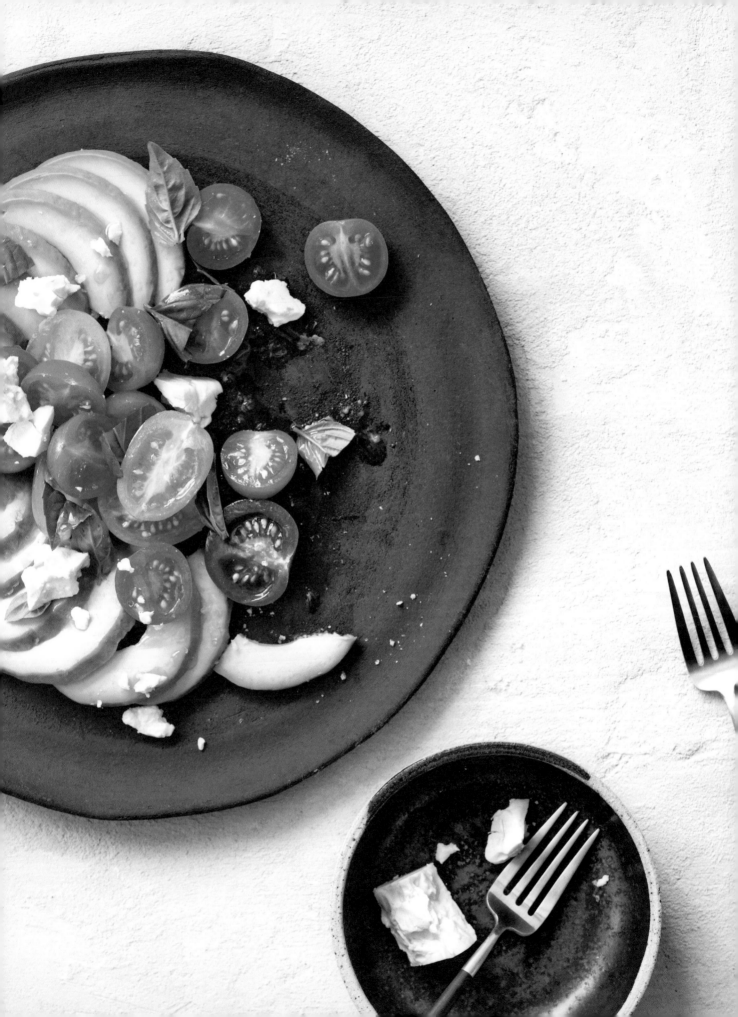

AVOCADO, TOMATO, FETA *and* BASIL SALAD

TOBIE I should really be asking my mum to write the introduction to this recipe, as I have blatantly stolen it from her. Mum, here's your credit – please release me from any trouble I may now be in! She has been making it for years and we just love it; it takes about 5 minutes to put together and tastes delicious. I like to use a few different varieties of heirloom tomatoes in this recipe – they look fantastic and give subtle flavour and texture variations that add extra interest, too.

200 g mixed tomatoes

sea salt and cracked black pepper

1 large avocado

100 g reduced-fat feta

handful of basil leaves, torn

1 tablespoon extra virgin olive oil

2 teaspoons balsamic vinegar

Cut the tomatoes into bite-sized pieces – if using cherry tomatoes, just cut them in half. Place in a bowl and season with salt and pepper.

Halve the avocado, remove the stone and use a spoon to scoop out the flesh in one piece or peel away the skin. Slice the flesh and arrange around the perimeter of a serving plate, slightly overlapping. Tip the tomato into the middle of the plate. Crumble over the feta, then tear the basil over and season with salt and pepper. Drizzle the olive oil and balsamic over the entire dish and serve right away.

SERVES: 4 AS A SIDE

	PER SERVE
ENERGY (KJ/CAL)	973/232
PROTEIN (G)	8
FAT (G)	21
SATURATED FAT (G)	6
CARBOHYDRATE (G)	1.5

EGGPLANT, BROCCOLI RABE *and* QUINOA

TOBIE We've been experimenting a lot with quinoa – this salad is a favourite combination.

1 large eggplant (aubergine), trimmed, cut into large chunks

2 tablespoons extra virgin olive oil

sea salt and cracked black pepper

¾ cup (150 g) quinoa

200 g broccoli rabe or broccolini, trimmed, cut into 3 cm pieces

2 cloves garlic, thinly sliced

¼ teaspoon smoked paprika

juice of 1 lemon

2 eggs, soft boiled, peeled and halved

Preheat the oven to 180°C. Line a baking tray with baking paper. Toss the eggplant with 2 teaspoons olive oil, salt and pepper, then scatter over the lined tray and bake for 30–40 minutes or until tender. Set aside.

Toast the quinoa in a heavy-based saucepan over medium heat, stirring constantly, for 2 minutes. Add 2 cups (500 ml) water and bring to the boil. Reduce the heat and hold at a simmer for 15 minutes. Turn off the heat and set aside, covered, for 5 minutes. Transfer to a large bowl and leave to cool in the fridge.

Bring a saucepan of salted water to the boil, add the broccoli rabe or broccolini and cook for 30 seconds, then drain and refresh under cold water.

Put the remaining olive oil in a small saucepan, add the garlic and warm over low–medium heat until it sizzles. Mix in the paprika; cool. Season to taste.

Dress the quinoa with the garlic oil, then add the lemon juice and mix well. Season to taste. Mix in the broccoli rabe or broccolini and cooked eggplant. Serve the salad with the soft-boiled eggs alongside.

SERVES: 4 AS A SIDE

	PER SERVE
ENERGY (KJ/CAL)	1154/276
PROTEIN (G)	11
FAT (G)	14
SATURATED FAT (G)	2.5
CARBOHYDRATE (G)	24

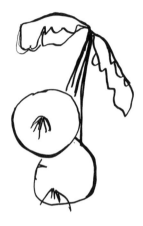

RAW BEET SALAD

SERVES: 6 AS A SIDE

	PER SERVE
ENERGY (KJ/CAL)	584/140
PROTEIN (G)	4.5
FAT (G)	11.5
SATURATED FAT (G)	3
CARBOHYDRATE (G)	3.5

3 beetroots (about 400 g in total)

1 tablespoon apple cider vinegar

2 tablespoons extra virgin olive oil

sea salt and cracked black pepper

big handful of flat-leaf parsley, roughly chopped

handful of mint leaves, thinly sliced

3 heaped tablespoons Seed and nut mix (see page 190)

80 g soft goat's cheese

TOBIE This salad is brilliant. It travels well and tastes just as good the next day, so it's perfect for picnics or to take to work. Planning ahead is vital if you want to keep up regular healthy eating, and making a veggie dish or salad that you can eat over the following days is a great idea. Just bear in mind that although robust ingredients like root vegetables hold up well when dressed, leaves and herbs do tend to wilt. So, if you are preparing a dish like this with a view to eating it later, pack the herbs separately and add them just before eating.

GEORGIA Beetroot, nuts and goat's cheese is an unbeatable combination. I sometimes add the beet leaves to this salad, too.

Wearing gloves to avoid staining your hands, top and tail the beetroots, peel using a potato peeler and then use a Japanese mandoline or the shredding disc on a food processor to shred them into a large bowl.

Put the vinegar, olive oil and a good pinch of both salt and pepper in a bowl and stir to combine.

Add the dressing to the beetroot, mix thoroughly and set aside for 10 minutes. Carefully fold through the parsley, mint and seed and nut mix, then crumble the goat's cheese over the top and serve right away.

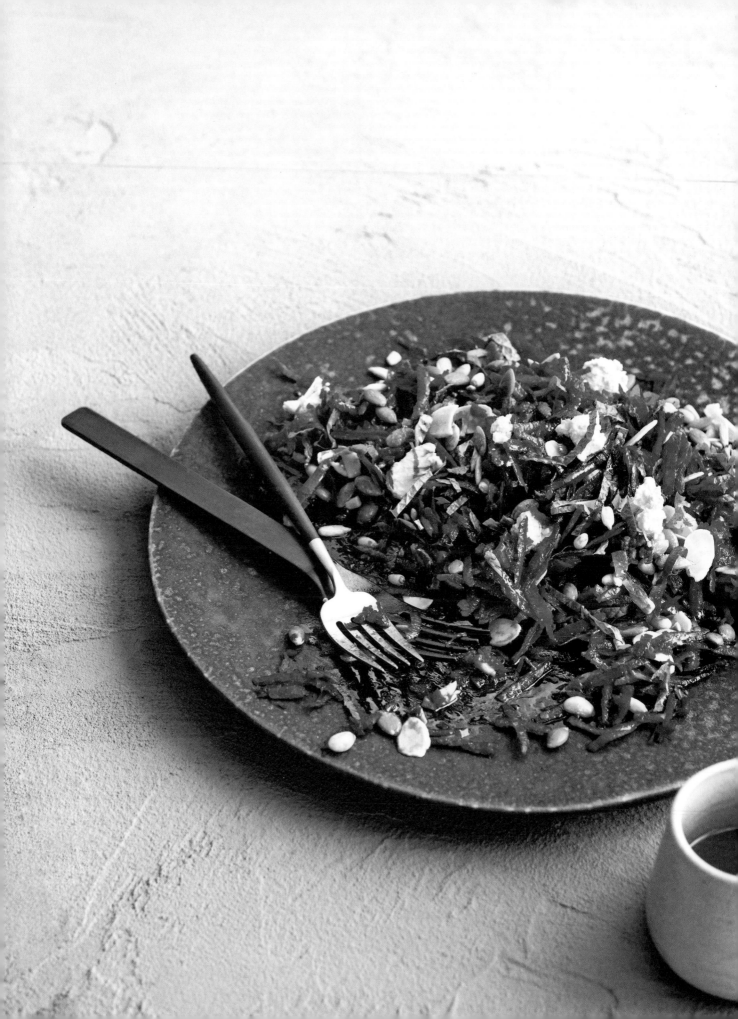

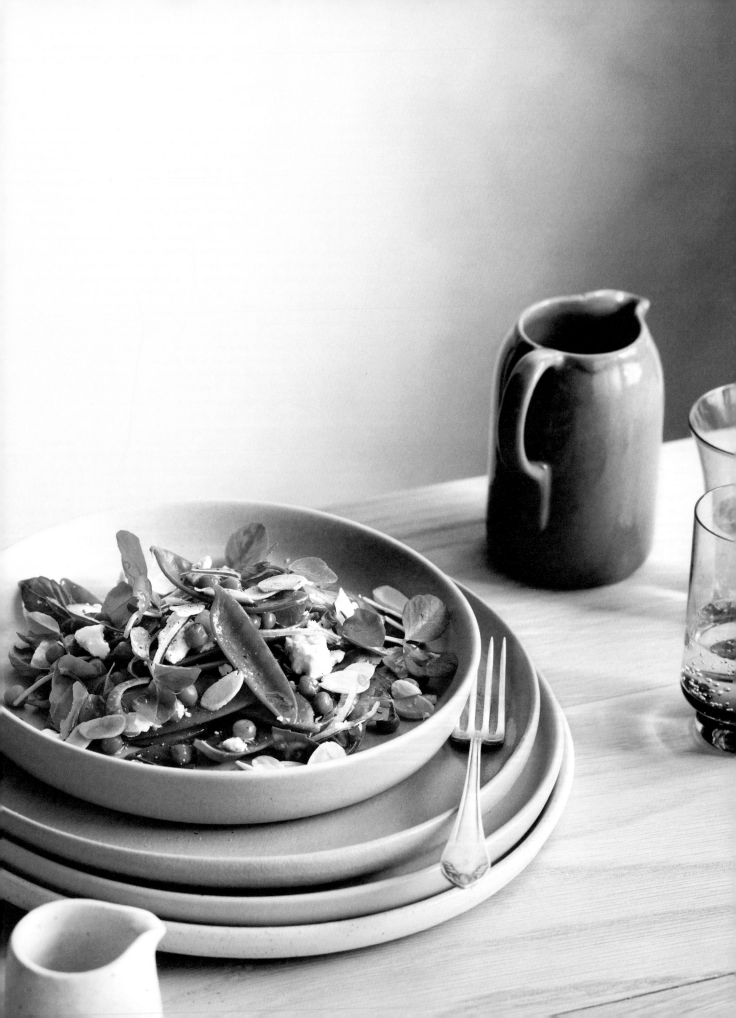

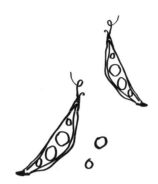

PEA, SNOWPEA, ALMOND and FETA SALAD

SERVES: 4 AS A SIDE

	PER SERVE
ENERGY (KJ/CAL)	801/192
PROTEIN (G)	9
FAT (G)	13
SATURATED FAT (G)	2.5
CARBOHYDRATE (G)	7.5

TOBIE There are a lot of nuts in this book. I used to eat a lot of chocolate, now I eat a lot of nuts! (Actually, I still eat chocolate, but more so nuts.) Anyway, the point is that very, very al dente snow peas and almonds are the bomb.

Bring a saucepan of water to the boil. Add the snowpeas and peas and blanch for 30–40 seconds or until bright green and tender crisp, then drain and refresh in cold water to stop the cooking process. Drain well.

Put the snowpeas, peas, onion, feta, almonds, basil, olive oil and vinegar in a large bowl and toss to combine. Season with salt and pepper, to taste. Carefully fold through the pea cress, rocket or watercress using your hands and serve right away.

150 g snowpeas (mange-tout), ends trimmed

150 g shelled fresh or thawed frozen peas

½ red onion, thinly sliced

50 g reduced-fat feta, crumbled

30 g flaked almonds, toasted

handful of basil leaves, roughly torn

1½ tablespoons extra virgin olive oil

2 teaspoons red wine vinegar

sea salt and cracked black pepper

handful of pea cress, rocket or picked watercress

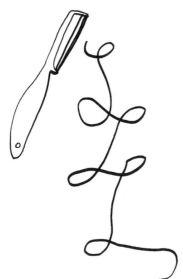

PARSNIP *and* CARROT SALAD

SERVES: 4 AS A SIDE

	PER SERVE
ENERGY (KJ/CAL)	724/173
PROTEIN (G)	3
FAT (G)	12.5
SATURATED FAT (G)	2
CARBOHYDRATE (G)	9.5

2 carrots (about 250 g)

2 parsnips (about 250 g)

2 tablespoons Seed and nut mix (see page 190)

handful of basil leaves, roughly torn

handful of mint leaves, roughly torn

MUSTARD DRESSING

2 tablespoons extra virgin olive oil

2 teaspoons gluten-free wholegrain mustard

finely grated zest and juice of ½ lemon

sea salt and cracked black pepper

TOBIE I first spotted Jamie Oliver doing ribbons of root vegetables for a salad and really liked the look of it, so I gave it a go and then started adding the flavours that come naturally to me, like basil and mint, and eventually the mustard dressing. The addition of the seed and nut mix not only brings goodness to the recipe, but a delightful texture as well.

Use a vegetable peeler to peel the skin from the carrots and parsnips and discard, then peel long strips from both vegetables and place in a large bowl.

To make the mustard dressing, put the olive oil, mustard and lemon zest and juice in a small bowl and use a fork or whisk to combine. Taste and season with salt and pepper.

Add the dressing to the carrot and parsnip, then add the seed and nut mix, basil and mint. Toss to combine, and serve.

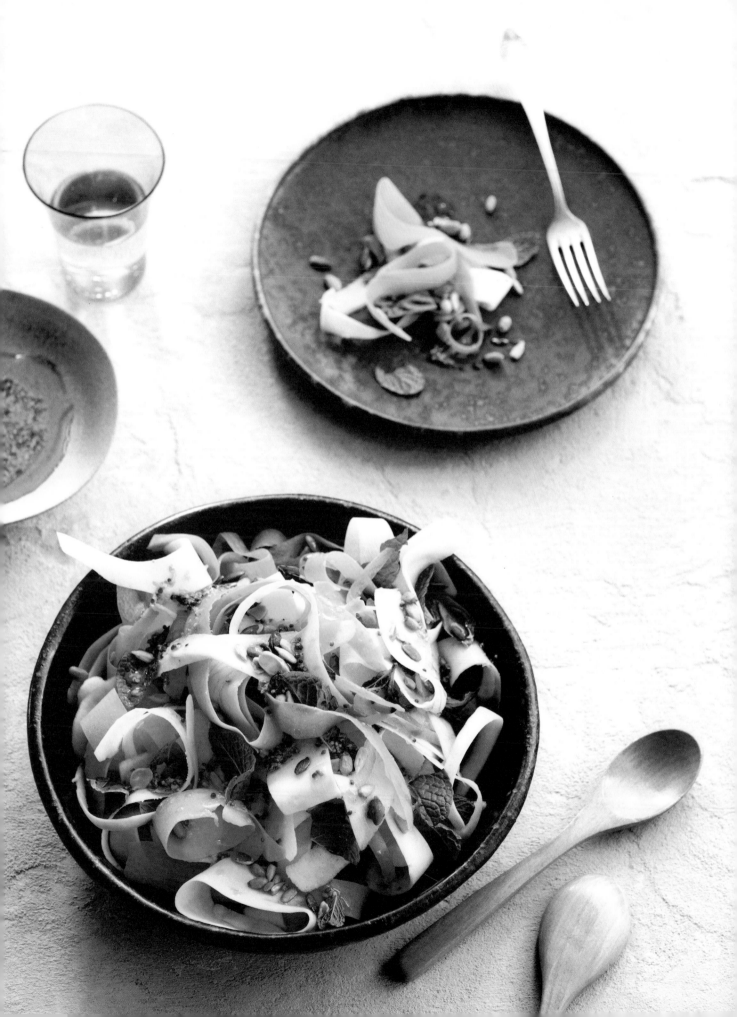

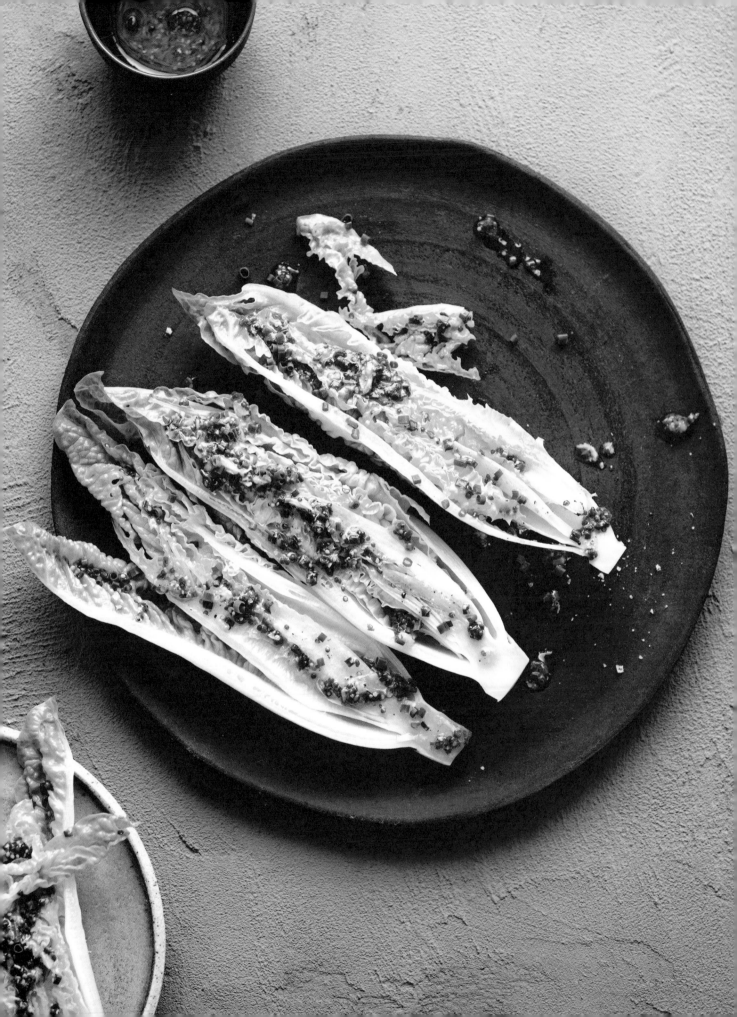

BABY COS SALAD

TOBIE At the risk of sounding fancy, when I was in Paris last year I was served a salad of the tiniest baby cos I have ever seen. They were so sweet and super crispy, and they were served with a beautiful red wine vinaigrette of sorts. Anyway, that's enough history – this is my version. If you can't get baby cos, just use the larger ones and take off the outer leaves, keeping them for another salad on another day.

2 tablespoons extra virgin olive oil

1 teaspoon gluten-free wholegrain mustard

1 teaspoon red wine vinegar

1 tablespoon finely chopped chives

1 small clove garlic, finely chopped or crushed

sea salt and cracked black pepper

6 baby cos lettuces or 3 larger cos lettuces

Put the olive oil, mustard, vinegar, chives, garlic and a good pinch of both salt and pepper in a small bowl and use a fork to whisk until combined.

Halve the baby lettuces, or quarter them if larger, and arrange on serving plates or a platter. Drizzle over the dressing and serve right away.

SERVES: 4–6 AS A SIDE

	PER SERVE (FOR 6)
ENERGY (KJ/CAL)	375/90
PROTEIN (G)	0.5
FAT (G)	9
SATURATED FAT (G)	1.5
CARBOHYDRATE (G)	0.5

FENNEL, PEAR and HAZELNUT SALAD

TOBIE This is really quick to make and I just love the combo of the hazelnuts with the sweetness of the pear and my favourite flavour, aniseed. If you are not a fennel fan you can swap it for celery or a leaf of some sort, like rocket.

2 bulbs baby fennel

2 ripe beurre bosc pears

1 tablespoon fresh lemon juice

1 tablespoon extra virgin olive oil

good handful of roasted and skinned hazelnuts, roughly chopped

sea salt and cracked black pepper

small handful of mint leaves, roughly torn

Trim the fennel bulbs and reserve the fronds. Thinly slice the fennel crossways using a knife, mandoline or vegetable peeler. Use a sharp knife to quarter the pears lengthways, remove the cores and slice into long thin strips.

Put the lemon juice and olive oil in a large bowl and give a little mix with a spoon. Add the fennel, pear and hazelnuts and season with salt and pepper. Fold in the mint and reserved fennel fronds and toss to combine. Serve right away.

SERVES: 4 AS A SIDE

	PER SERVE
ENERGY (KJ/CAL)	640/153
PROTEIN (G)	2
FAT (G)	7
SATURATED FAT (G)	1
CARBOHYDRATE (G)	18.5

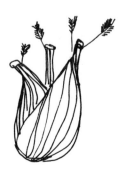

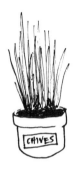

SMOKED TROUT, ROASTED BEETS, HORSERADISH *and* CRESS SALAD

SERVES: 4 AS A SIDE

	PER SERVE
ENERGY (KJ/CAL)	927/221
PROTEIN (G)	10
FAT (G)	16
SATURATED FAT (G)	3
CARBOHYDRATE (G)	8

1 bunch baby beetroots,
ends trimmed

¼ cup (60 ml) extra virgin olive oil

sea salt and cracked black pepper

2 teaspoons freshly grated
horseradish, or to taste

2 teaspoons balsamic vinegar

small handful of chives,
finely chopped

150 g smoked trout or Rainbow
trout baked in salt (see page 99)

100 g picked watercress,
pea cress or rocket

TOBIE The trick to writing this book has been taking combinations of ingredients I know work well, like smoked trout, horseradish and beets, and tweaking them so that the likes of Georgia and Donna Aston approve. This dish makes a perfect starter or a great salad for lunch and you can swap the trout for smoked salmon, prosciutto or bresaola. You can use creamed horseradish if fresh horseradish is not available or if you simply prefer the flavour (if you don't eat gluten, check the label to make sure it's gluten free).

Preheat the oven to 200°C. Line a baking tray with baking paper.

Plunge the beetroots into a bowl of cold water and use a scrubbing brush to clean them thoroughly. Drain and rinse, then transfer to a bowl, add 1 tablespoon of the olive oil, season with salt and pepper and toss to coat well. Place the beetroots on the lined tray and bake for 30–40 minutes or until they can be easily pierced with a sharp knife. Remove from the oven and leave to cool before slicing each beetroot in half lengthways.

Combine the remaining olive oil, horseradish, vinegar and a good pinch of both salt and pepper in a small bowl.

Pop the beetroot into a bowl and pour over half of the dressing, then add the chives and mix gently to combine.

Break up the trout into bite-sized pieces and arrange on a serving platter with the dressed beets. Gently coat the cress or rocket with the remaining dressing and scatter over the trout and beets. Finish with a grind of pepper and a little more horseradish, if you wish. Serve.

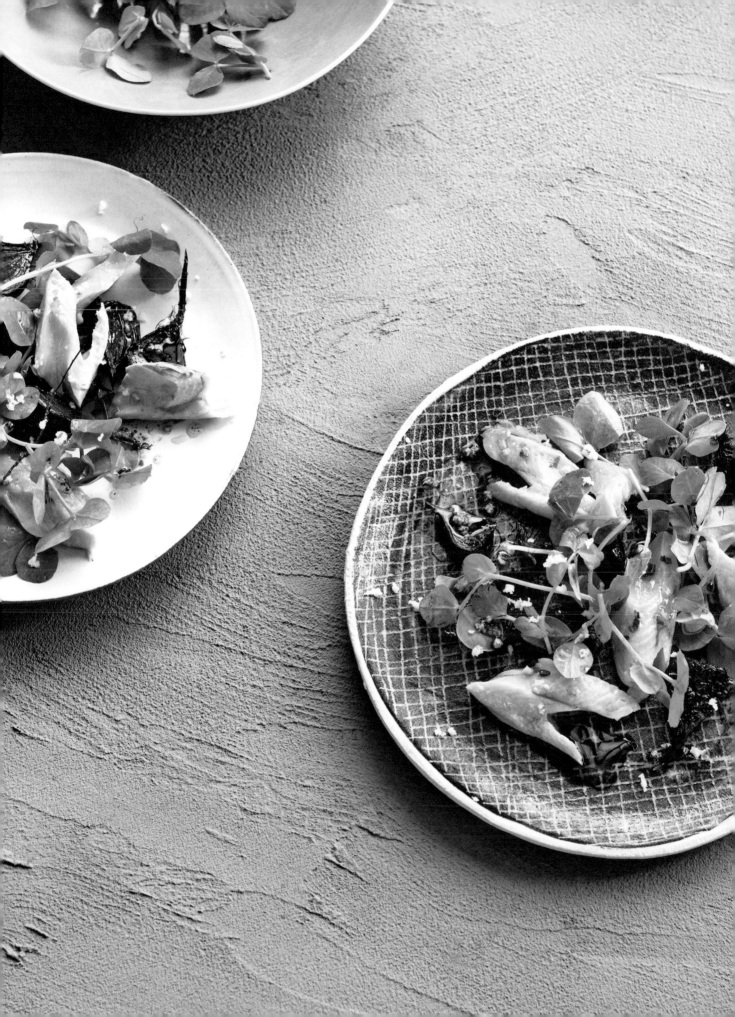

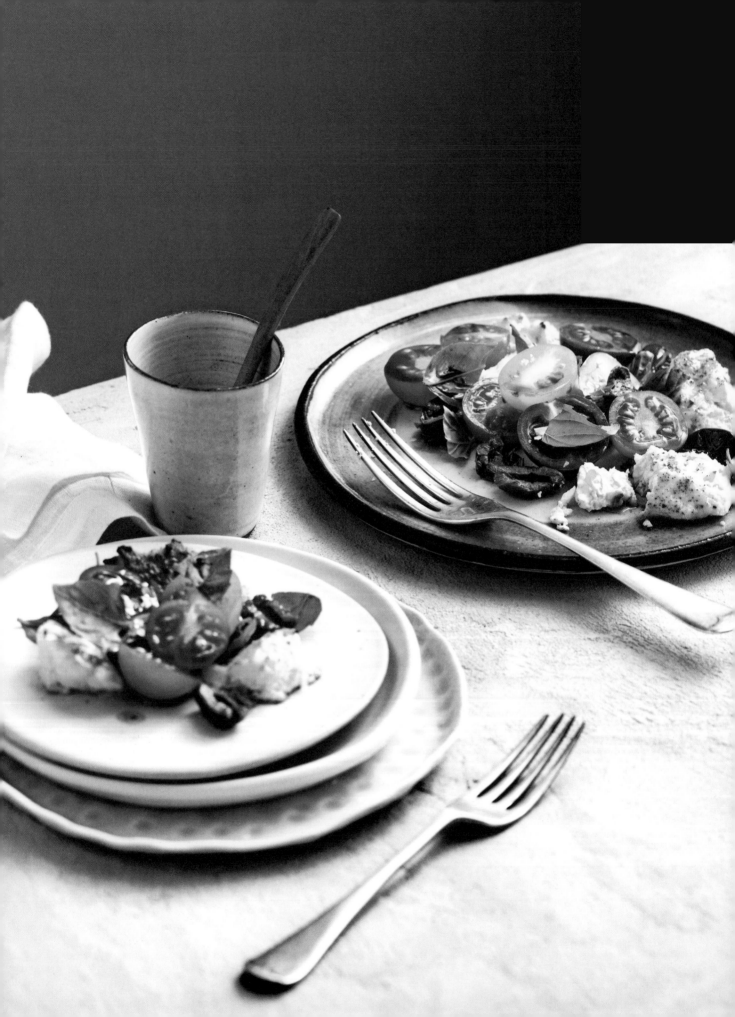

TOMATO, RICOTTA, BASIL *and* BALSAMIC SALAD

TOBIE One of my favourite things in this world is the famous *insalata caprese* (an Italian salad of tomato, mozzarella and basil). This version is a little friendlier on the hips and uses baked ricotta, which has a beautiful texture. You can use any tomatoes you like here, but you'll get the best result when they're nice and ripe, and if you can use a mixture of varieties the salad will look even prettier.

Preheat the oven to 180°C.

Line a baking tray with baking paper and drizzle about a teaspoon of olive oil over the paper. Break the ricotta into large clumps, each about the size of an oddly shaped golf ball, and place on the prepared tray. Season with salt, pepper and chilli flakes, then drizzle with more olive oil (about a teaspoon will do). Bake for 10–15 minutes or until the ricotta starts to turn a lovely golden colour. Remove from the oven and set aside to cool.

Thickly slice the tomatoes, or halve them if using cherry tomatoes, and place in a bowl. Tear in the basil and add the olives, 2 tablespoons olive oil and vinegar. Season with salt and pepper and toss very gently to combine.

Divide the tomato mixture among serving plates or place on a large platter, add the baked ricotta and serve.

SERVES: 4 AS A SIDE

	PER SERVE
ENERGY (KJ/CAL)	1356/324
PROTEIN (G)	10.5
FAT (G)	27
SATURATED FAT (G)	8
CARBOHYDRATE (G)	8

2 tablespoons extra virgin olive oil, plus extra, for drizzling

400 g firm fresh ricotta

sea salt and cracked black pepper

pinch of dried chilli flakes

500 g ripe tomatoes

handful of basil leaves (about 25)

150 g pitted black olives, halved

1 tablespoon balsamic vinegar

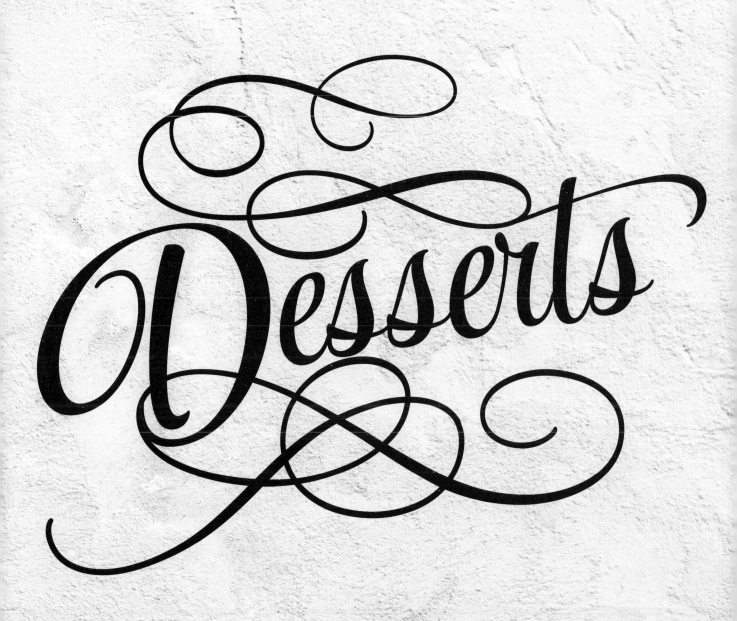

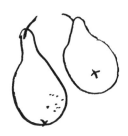

BAKED PEARS *with* SAFFRON, CINNAMON *and* VANILLA

SERVES: 4

	PER SERVE
ENERGY (KJ/CAL)	684/164
PROTEIN (G)	3
FAT (G)	4
SATURATED FAT (G)	0.5
CARBOHYDRATE (G)	27

4 firm beurre bosc pears, peeled

400 ml water or white wine
(or a combination of both)

1 tablespoon pure maple syrup

long strip of orange zest

1 cinnamon stick

1 vanilla bean, split lengthways
and seeds scraped

pinch of saffron threads

4 tablespoons low-fat plain
Greek-style yoghurt

2 tablespoons Seed and nut mix
(see page 190)

TOBIE Cinnamon, vanilla and sugar is a classic combination, but you can get a similar result using maple syrup and the natural sweetness of the pears to replace the refined sugar. Of course, for many years I would have added butter to the mix as well, but it really doesn't need it and leaving it out reduces the fat content of this dish dramatically. You can make this without the maple syrup too, and it's still a beautiful dessert. I simply peel the pears here, but feel free to core and/or halve them if you like. This will reduce the cooking time, so use a small knife to test them – when it pierces the pear easily, they're cooked.

Preheat the oven to 180°C. Trim the base of the pears, just a few millimetres, to make them flat so they can stand upright.

Put the water or wine, maple syrup, orange zest, cinnamon stick, vanilla seeds and pod, and saffron in a deep ovenproof saucepan and bring to a gentle simmer over low heat.

Add the pears to the pan, standing upright if possible, and carefully place in the oven. Cook the pears, basting with the cooking liquid every 10 minutes or so, for 40–50 minutes or until tender. If your pears are not standing upright, turn them every now and then so they cook evenly. Remove from the oven and set aside to cool.

Serve the pears with some of the cooking liquid spooned over, a dollop of yoghurt and the seed and nut mix scattered the top.

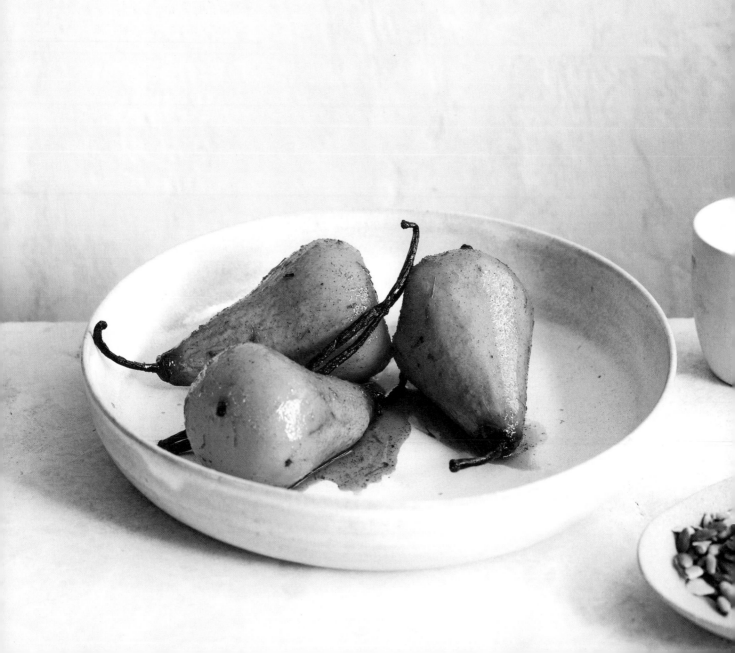

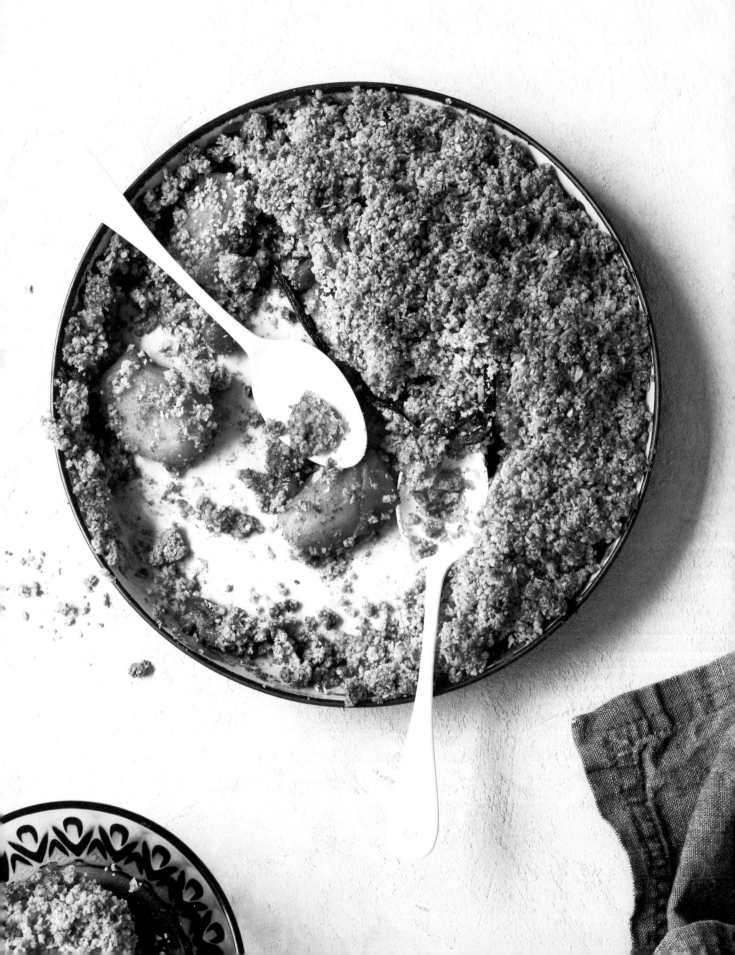

APPLE CRUMBLE

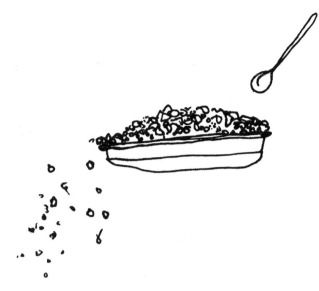

TOBIE Ask me to write one hundred low-carb savoury recipes without refined sugar or gluten, and I can make it happen with some trial and error, but desserts are a bit more complicated. I wanted to use ingredients that are natural and easy to find, and discovered that quinoa flakes are an excellent option. I hadn't tried using them in desserts before, but now I'm a convert. Thanks to everyone at Prahran Health Foods for the advice.

GEORGIA Dessert isn't really part of my diet plan, but look at this crumble! The refined sugar and butter are gone, yet it still tastes divine. Since this isn't an everyday sort of thing, I might even add a small bit of cream on top (for added calcium, of course!).

Preheat the oven to 180°C.

Pop the apple wedges, 1 cup (250 ml) water, orange zest, vanilla seeds and pod, cinnamon, nutmeg and sultanas into a large heavy-based saucepan. Cook over low heat, stirring occasionally, for 20 minutes or until the apple wedges are tender.

Meanwhile, to make the crumble, put all the ingredients in a food processor and pulse until the mixture resembles coarse breadcrumbs.

Spread the apple mixture evenly over the base of a round or square baking dish, about 5 cm deep. Scatter the crumble over the top, making sure it's an even thickness, then bake for 30 minutes or until the crumble is golden. Serve.

SERVES: 6

	PER SERVE
ENERGY (KJ/CAL)	1514/362
PROTEIN (G)	5.5
FAT (G)	14
SATURATED FAT (G)	6.5
CARBOHYDRATE (G)	51

6 pink lady apples, peeled, cored and cut into 8 wedges each

finely grated zest of 1 orange

1 vanilla bean, split lengthways and seeds scraped

1 teaspoon ground cinnamon

1 teaspoon ground nutmeg

½ cup (80 g) sultanas

CRUMBLE

1½ cups (165 g) quinoa flakes

1 teaspoon vanilla extract

2 tablespoons pure maple syrup

2 tablespoons virgin coconut oil

½ cup (50 g) walnuts

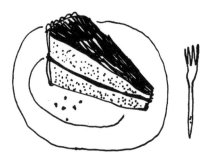

VEGAN CHOCOLATE CAKE

SERVES: 8–10

	PER SERVE (FOR 10)
ENERGY (KJ/CAL)	1913/458
PROTEIN (G)	4.5
FAT (G)	27.5
SATURATED FAT (G)	8.5
CARBOHYDRATE (G)	47.5

extra virgin olive oil, for greasing

½ cup (50 g) walnuts

1⅔ cups (210 g) gluten-free
self-raising flour

½ cup (50 g) gluten-free
cocoa powder

1 teaspoon bicarbonate of soda

pinch of sea salt

½ cup (125 ml) extra virgin olive oil

½ cup (125 ml) agave syrup

½ cup (125 ml) pure maple syrup

sliced strawberries or roughly
chopped walnuts, to serve

CASHEW CREAM

¾ cup (115 g) unsalted raw cashews

1 teaspoon fresh lemon juice

¼ teaspoon apple cider vinegar

pinch of sea salt

FROSTING

95 g gluten-free dark chocolate,
chopped and melted

2 tablespoons melted virgin
coconut oil

1 teaspoon vanilla extract

finely grated zest of ½ orange or
mandarin (optional)

TOBIE If you'd told me, 10 or even 20 years ago, that I would one day write a recipe for a vegan chocolate cake, I'd have given you the 'Can I speak to the manager?' expression. But here it is, and I have to say it tastes beautiful. Try pouring just a little whiskey over the cake before serving.

To make the cashew cream, pop the cashews in a bowl, add enough water to cover them completely and set aside for about 4 hours to soak.

Preheat the oven to 180°C. Grease a 25 cm springform cake tin with a little extra virgin olive oil and line the base with baking paper. Grease the paper.

Drain and rinse the soaked cashews, then place in a food processor with ½ cup (125 ml) water, the lemon juice, vinegar and salt. Process until smooth and thick. Transfer to a bowl, then wash and dry the food processor.

Blitz the walnuts in the food processor until finely chopped, with a consistency similar to almond meal. Add the gluten-free flour, cocoa powder, bicarbonate of soda and salt and pulse a few times, until well combined.

Place the olive oil, agave syrup, maple syrup, cashew cream and ½ cup (125 ml) water in a bowl and use an electric mixer on low speed to beat until combined. Add the dry ingredients and beat until thoroughly combined. Pour into the prepared tin and bake for 35 minutes or until the top of the cake springs back when touched and a skewer inserted into the centre of the cake comes out clean. Transfer to a wire rack and leave for 10 minutes, then remove from the tin and allow to cool completely.

Meanwhile, to make the frosting, put the melted chocolate, coconut oil, vanilla and orange or mandarin zest, if using, in a bowl and use hand-held electric beaters to beat until thick and creamy. Cover and place in the fridge for about 5 minutes to firm up to a spreadable consistency.

Remove the cooled cake from the tin, place on a serving plate and use a spatula to cover with the frosting. Serve with the strawberries or walnuts.

TIP The cake will keep for up to 2 days in an airtight container.

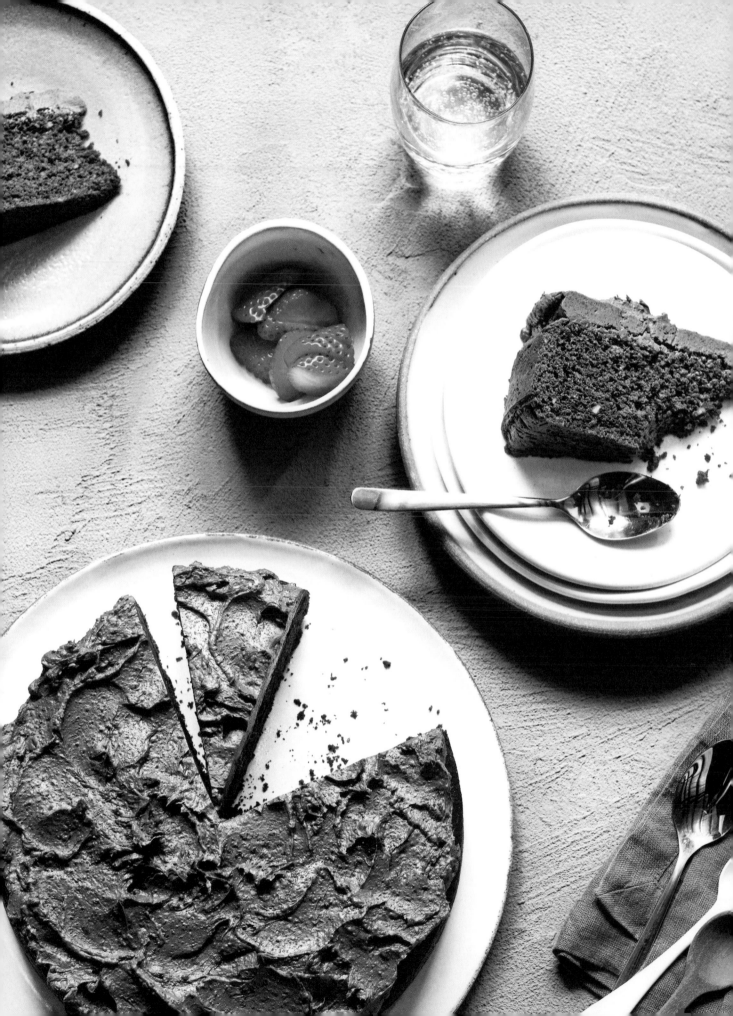

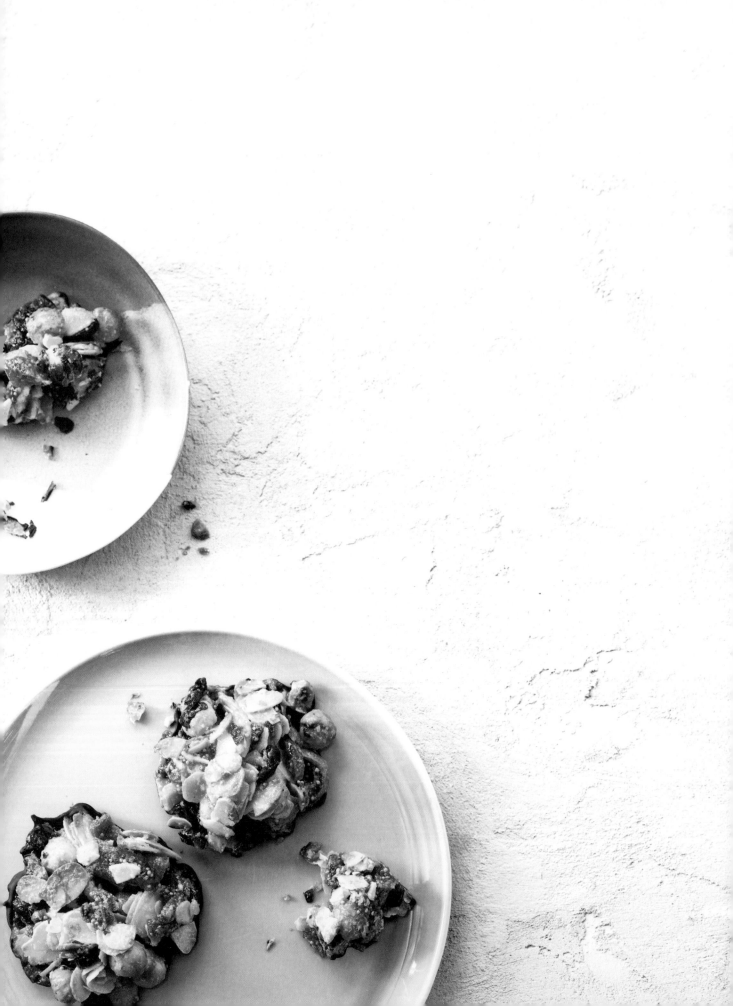

FLORENTINES

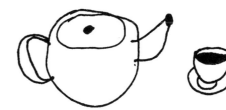

TOBIE I've always enjoyed a good florentine. My parents used to take me down to Acland Street in Melbourne when I was a little boy and a florentine would always land in my hand at some point. They usually contain candied fruits, sugar and butter, so they're not exactly a healthy treat and you'd probably have to go for a pretty long run to break even after you eat one. However, the only sugar in this recipe is in the form of brown rice syrup (also known as rice malt syrup) and the natural sugars in the dried fruit, and there's no butter. So while they're not on par with carrot sticks, they're much better for you than a traditional florentine.

Preheat the oven to 180°C. Line 2 baking trays with baking paper.

Scatter the hazelnuts over one of the lined trays and the flaked almonds over the other. Bake until the nuts are just starting to colour, then remove and set aside to cool (the almonds will need less time than the hazelnuts). Once cooled, tip the hazelnuts onto a clean tea towel and rub vigorously to remove the skins. Place the nuts in a bowl with the cranberries and figs.

Put the rice syrup and orange zest in a small saucepan and warm over low heat for 1 minute, then add the almond meal and stir for 1 minute, until combined and the mixture thickens slightly. Pour the syrup mixture into the bowl with the nuts and fruit and stir until thoroughly combined.

Line a large baking tray with baking paper. Spoon heaped tablespoons of the mixture onto the tray, allowing 4 cm between each for spreading. Use slightly wet fingertips to bunch the ingredients together to make little rounds. Bake the florentines for 15 minutes or until they are light golden. Leave on the tray for 10 minutes, then transfer to a wire rack and set aside to cool completely.

Meanwhile, melt the chocolate in a heatproof bowl over a saucepan of simmering water (make sure the water doesn't touch the base of the bowl). Use a metal spoon to spread the melted chocolate over the base of each florentine. Place, chocolate side up, on a wire rack. When the chocolate has almost set, gently drag a fork over it to make lines. Leave to set completely.

TIP The florentines will keep for up to 2 weeks in an airtight container.

MAKES: 12

	PER FLORENTINE
ENERGY (KJ/CAL)	940/225
PROTEIN (G)	4
FAT (G)	12.5
SATURATED FAT (G)	2.5
CARBOHYDRATE (G)	24.5

60 g hazelnuts

¾ cup (60 g) flaked almonds

50 g sweetened dried cranberries, roughly chopped

80 g dried figs, roughly chopped

150 g brown rice syrup

finely grated zest of ½ orange

20 g almond meal

150 g gluten-free dark chocolate, broken into pieces

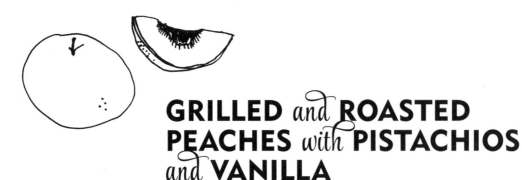

GRILLED and ROASTED PEACHES with PISTACHIOS and VANILLA

SERVES: 4

	PER SERVE
ENERGY (KJ/CAL)	1012/242
PROTEIN (G)	5.5
FAT (G)	8
SATURATED FAT (G)	1
CARBOHYDRATE (G)	28.5

4 freestone peaches, halved and stones removed

1 teaspoon extra virgin olive oil

1 cup (250 ml) white wine

¼ cup (60 ml) pure maple syrup

1 vanilla bean, split lengthways and seeds scraped

1 star anise

50 g pistachio kernels, lightly bashed with a mortar and pestle

low-fat plain Greek-style yoghurt, to serve

TOBIE Peaches are beautifully sweet just as they are and therefore we really don't need to do much to them. I like to give them a little stint on the grill for an ever-so-slightly charred flavour, then a turn in the oven to make them a little softer and even sweeter. Freestone (or slipstone) peaches, as the name implies, are the ones where the stones come away easily from the flesh. In this type of dish they look much better (and are much easier to work with), so try to get them if you can. The other type of peach is called clingstone.

Preheat the oven to 180°C and line a shallow baking dish with baking paper. Heat a chargrill pan over low heat.

Use a pastry brush to brush the cut surface of each peach with olive oil. Place a piece of baking paper on the chargrill pan, then put the peaches flesh-side down on the paper and cook for about 3 minutes. Carefully lift up each peach and rotate it just a little, then cook for a further 3 minutes, until the peaches have a lovely lattice pattern of grill marks. Use a spatula to transfer the peaches to the lined dish, cut side up.

Put the white wine, maple syrup, vanilla seeds and pod, and star anise in a small saucepan over medium heat. Bring to the boil, then immediately reduce the heat and hold at a simmer for 1 minute.

Pour the syrup over the hot peaches, then bake for 15 minutes. Remove from the oven and scatter the pistachios over the peaches, then bake for a further 10 minutes. Serve warm with yoghurt.

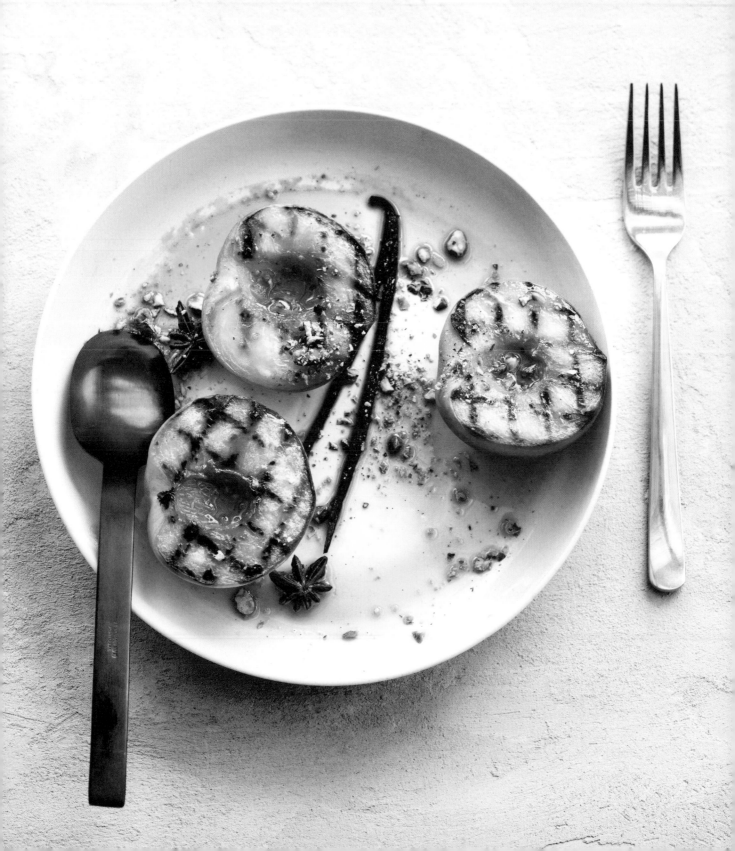

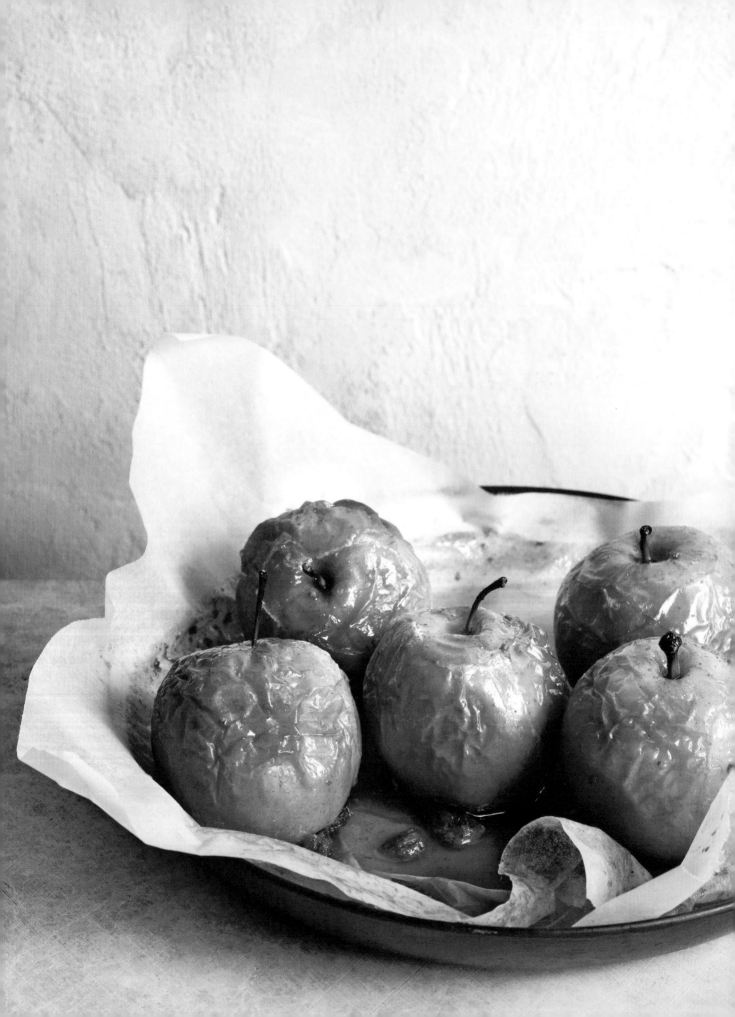

BAKED APPLES *with* RUM, RAISINS *and* PECANS

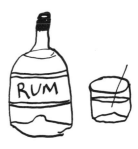

SERVES: 6

	PER SERVE
ENERGY (KJ/CAL)	1556/372
PROTEIN (G)	4
FAT (G)	12.5
SATURATED FAT (G)	1
CARBOHYDRATE (G)	52.5

TOBIE This recipe is really gorgeous and if you're in the mood for something indulgent, it's also delicious served with vanilla ice-cream. You can add some finely grated citrus zest to the filling to give it an extra pop of flavour – orange and mandarin work particularly well. You can use any variety of apple here, but I've found royal gala works a treat.

¾ cup (110 g) raisins

75 ml rum

105 g pecan halves, roughly chopped

1½ teaspoons ground cinnamon

large pinch of ground cardamom

6 apples

135 g honey

low-fat plain Greek-style yoghurt, to serve

Preheat the oven to 180°C. Line a 5 cm-deep baking dish with baking paper.

Put the raisins and rum in a small bowl and set aside for at least 30 minutes. The raisins will soften and soak up the flavour of the rum.

Add the pecans and spices to the soaked raisins and stir to combine.

Use an apple corer to remove the cores from the apples. (If you have an old-fashioned corer that looks a bit like a curved, double-edged knife, work from the bottom of each apple to about halfway up and leave the top of the cores intact. If you have a modern corer, with a serrated circular top, just remove the cores entirely. I use a teaspoon to hollow out the apples a little bit more so they will be able to hold a decent amount of filling.) Discard the apple cores and seeds.

Use your fingers to stuff the filling into the apples, packing it in so that it's quite dense. Place the apples in the lined dish, standing upright.

Stir the honey and 450 ml water in a small saucepan over low–medium heat until warm and combined. Pour over the apples, then bake for 1 hour, basting the apples with the honey mixture every 10 minutes or so. Set aside to cool slightly before serving with a dollop of yoghurt.

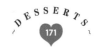

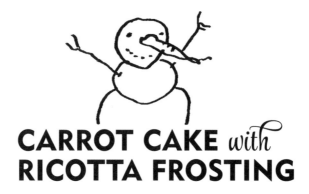

CARROT CAKE *with* RICOTTA FROSTING

	PER SERVE (FOR 10)
ENERGY (KJ/CAL)	1775/425
PROTEIN (G)	12
FAT (G)	32.5
SATURATED FAT (G)	8.5
CARBOHYDRATE (G)	19.5

olive oil, for greasing

500 g carrots, coarsely grated

2½ cups (300 g) almond meal

1 vanilla bean, split lengthways and seeds scraped

2 teaspoons gluten-free baking powder

1 teaspoon ground cinnamon

1 teaspoon fennel seeds, toasted and ground

good pinch of ground nutmeg

finely grated zest of 1 orange

150 ml pure maple syrup

70 ml melted virgin coconut oil or cold-pressed extra virgin olive oil

3 eggs, lightly whisked

¾ cup (75 g) roughly chopped walnuts, to garnish

RICOTTA FROSTING

200 g low-fat ricotta

30 g honey

TOBIE Carrot cake has been a favourite of mine for many years, so I couldn't imagine giving it up. This healthy take on it is just as moist, light and flavoursome as the original.

GEORGIA I always thought that without the divine cream cheese frosting carrot cake might lose its appeal, but I can happily report that's not the case! This whipped ricotta and honey frosting is an excellent alternative and can be used to top other cakes, too.

Preheat the oven to 180°C. Grease a round 20 cm springform cake tin using a little olive oil, then line with baking paper and lightly grease the paper. (I am a bit paranoid about things getting stuck, so I grease the paper as well just to be on the safe side, but if you don't want to that's up to you.)

Put the carrot, almond meal, vanilla seeds, baking powder, cinnamon, fennel seeds, nutmeg and orange zest in a large bowl and mix with a wooden spoon until well combined. Add the maple syrup, coconut or olive oil and eggs and mix until thoroughly combined. (Alternatively, mix in a stand mixer using the paddle attachment.)

Pour the mixture into the prepared tin and bake for 1 hour or until a skewer inserted into the centre of the cake comes out clean and the centre is firm to the touch. If the top starts to brown too much, cover it loosely with foil. Transfer to a wire rack and leave for 10 minutes before removing from the tin, then set aside to cool completely.

To make the ricotta frosting, place the ricotta and honey in a bowl and whip with a balloon whisk until smooth and slightly aerated. Cover with plastic film and place in the fridge until needed.

Use a spatula to spread the ricotta frosting over the cooled cake. Scatter the chopped walnuts over the cake and it's time to eat!

TIP The cake will keep for up to 2 days in an airtight container in the fridge.

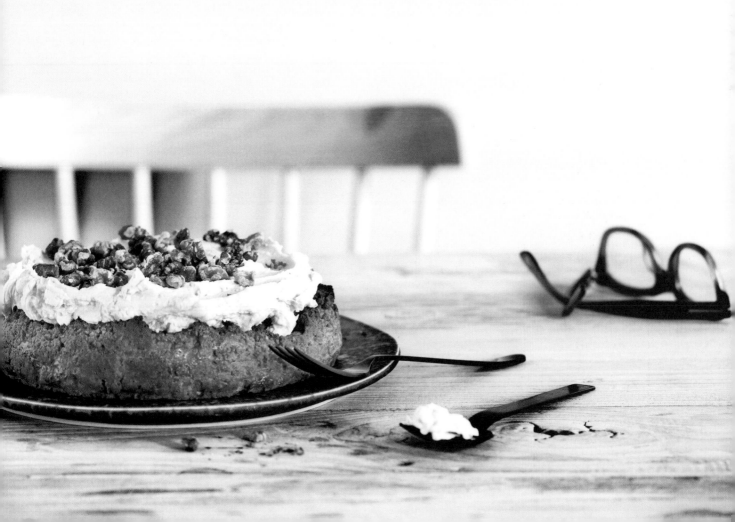

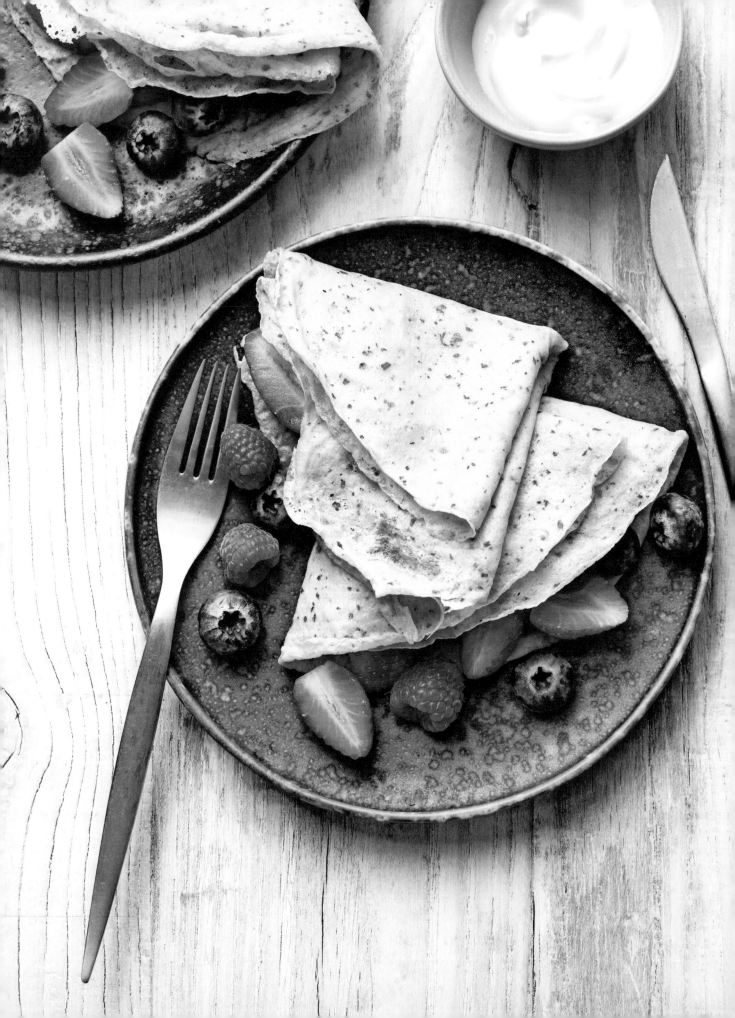

ALMOND CREPES *with* BERRIES *and* YOGHURT

MAKES: 8

	PER FILLED CREPE
ENERGY (KJ/CAL)	794/190
PROTEIN (G)	7.5
FAT (G)	10
SATURATED FAT (G)	2.5
CARBOHYDRATE (G)	16.5

TOBIE I've written a few recipes for crepes in my time, but here's the new healthy version, sans creme fraiche, gluten and refined sugar, and welcoming the beautiful flavour of almond milk.

Use a balloon whisk to whisk the eggs, almond milk, ⅓ cup (80 ml) water, honey or maple syrup, and salt in a large bowl until combined. Add the almond meal and flour and whisk until the mixture is smooth and well combined. Cover with plastic film and leave to rest in the fridge for at least 20 minutes before using.

Heat a 20 cm non-stick frying pan over medium heat. Dab a little coconut oil on a piece of paper towel and rub over the pan so it's evenly greased. Pour a ladleful of batter into the pan and immediately jiggle the pan to distribute the batter evenly over the base. If you have too much mixture in the pan, just tilt the pan over the bowl of batter and let the excess run back into the bowl. When the crepe is starting to brown underneath, flip it and repeat to cook the other side. Transfer the crepe to an upside-down plate (this is a great trick I learned as an apprentice – the crepes don't stick to the plate and sweat the way they do when it's right-side up) and cover with a clean tea towel. Repeat to cook the rest of the crepes, stacking them on the plate as you go and greasing the pan as necessary.

Place a crepe on a serving plate and put a mound of berries in one quarter, then fold in half and half again to make a quarter-sized crepe. Repeat to fill the remaining crepes. Serve topped with a dollop of yoghurt.

5 eggs

150 ml almond milk

2 teaspoons honey or pure maple syrup

pinch of sea salt

50 g almond meal

100 g gluten-free plain flour

virgin coconut oil, for frying

300 g mixed berries (fresh or thawed frozen)

low-fat plain Greek-style yoghurt, to serve

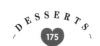

DATE, CHOCOLATE and MACADAMIA BITES

MAKES: ABOUT 25

	PER BITE
ENERGY (KJ/CAL)	666/159
PROTEIN (G)	1.5
FAT (G)	10.5
SATURATED FAT (G)	4.5
CARBOHYDRATE (G)	14.5

450 g dark chocolate, broken into pieces

150 g unsalted raw macadamias

100 g pitted dates, roughly chopped

40 g desiccated coconut

TOBIE I have to admit I've got a bit of a sweet tooth and, given the opportunity, would eat chocolate for breakfast. These little bites hit the spot when I have a craving for something sweet. I've used macadamia nuts, but you could use just about any nut instead. The same goes for the dried fruit.

GEORGIA I don't think I could give up chocolate completely, but I've done a good job on cutting down from what I used to eat. One of these, every now and then, is just the right kind of indulgence.

Melt the chocolate in a large heatproof bowl over a saucepan of simmering water (make sure the water doesn't touch the base of the bowl).

Meanwhile, pop the macadamias into a food processor and pulse briefly a couple of times just to break them up a bit. Transfer 100 g of the chopped nuts to a bowl. Pulse the remaining nuts a few more times until they have the consistency of coarse breadcrumbs, then set aside.

When the chocolate is melted, remove the bowl from the pan and use a large metal spoon to fold through the dates, coconut and 100 g of the chopped macadamias until thoroughly combined.

Line a tray with baking paper. Spoon clumps of the mixture onto the lined tray, in mounds about half the size of a golf ball. Scatter over the finely chopped macadamias, then place in the fridge for about an hour to set.

TIP These delicious little morsels will keep for up to a month in an airtight container in a cool, dark cupboard or the fridge if the weather is warm.

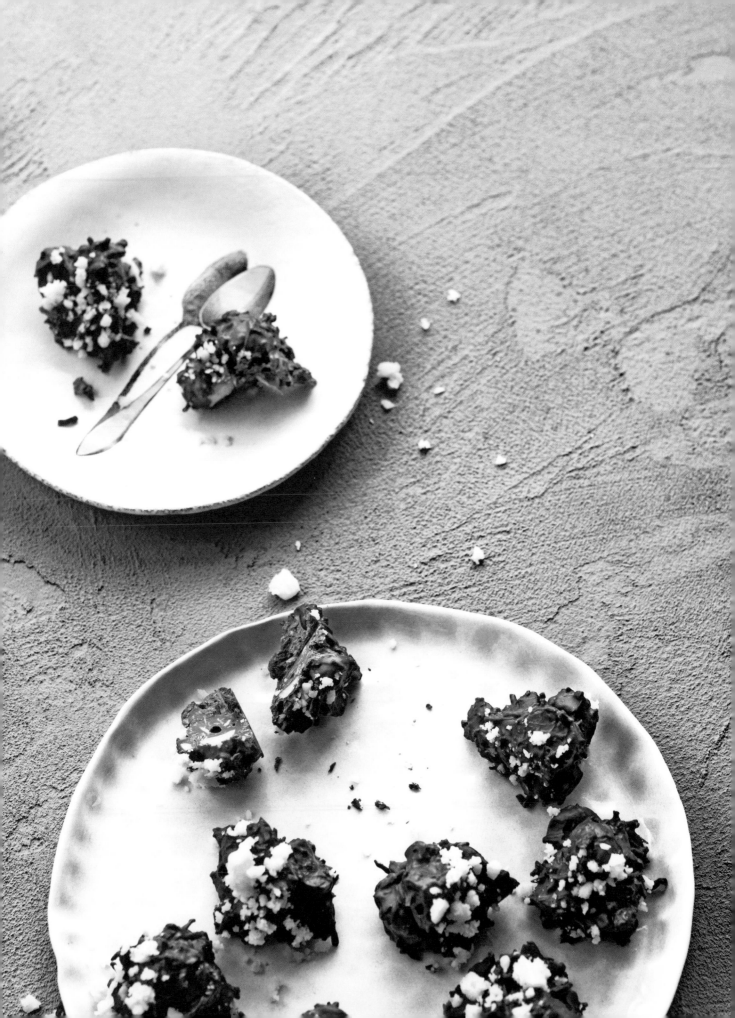

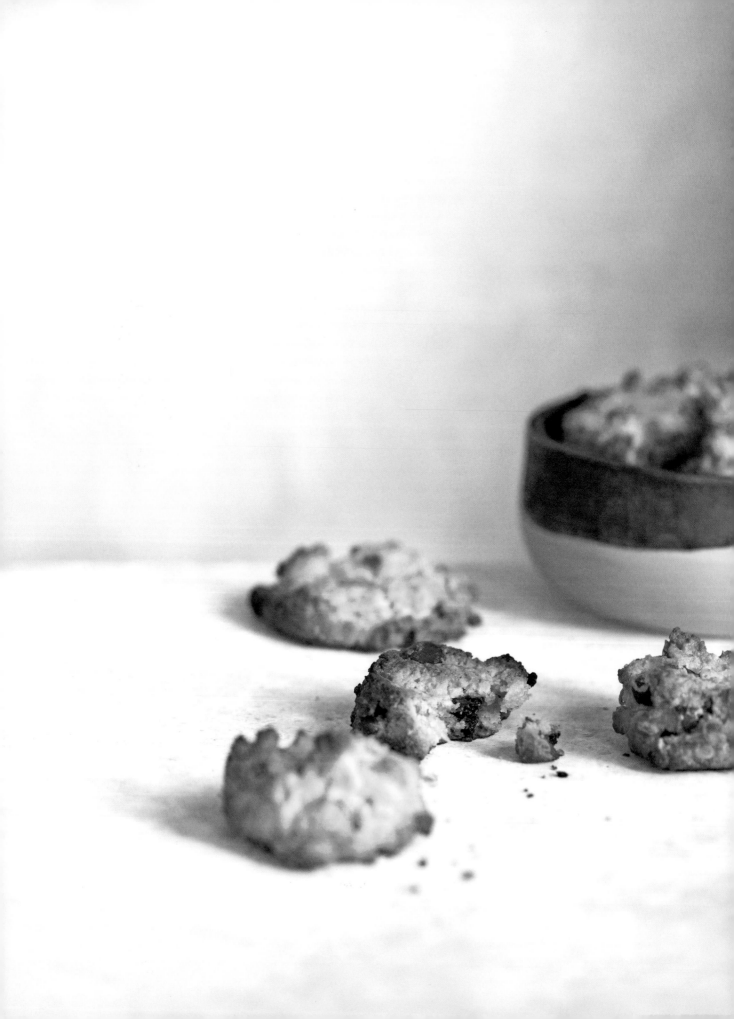

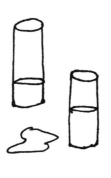
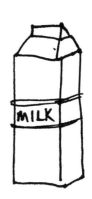

MACADAMIA BUTTER and CHOC CHIP COOKIES

This recipe started out as peanut butter and choc chip cookies, but I ran out of peanuts so I used my macadamia butter instead and the outcome was smiles for miles. These will keep for up to a week, but there's no chance of that happening – on the photo shoot they didn't even last until they had cooled!

Preheat the oven to 200°C. Line a large baking tray with baking paper.

Combine the quinoa flakes, almond meal and flour in a large bowl.

Use the paddle attachment on a stand mixer to mix the macadamia butter, brown rice syrup, grated apple and vanilla extract on low speed until combined. (This can also be done in a large bowl with a wooden spoon.) Fold through the quinoa mixture, followed by the choc chips.

Spoon tablespoons of the mixture onto the lined tray, leaving about 2 cm between each to allow for spreading and pressing them down to flatten slightly. Bake the cookies for 20–25 minutes or until browned on top.

Remove and cool on the tray for 5 minutes before transferring to a wire rack to cool completely.

TIP The cookies will keep for up to a week in an airtight container.

MAKES 15

	PER COOKIE
ENERGY (KJ/CAL)	758/181
PROTEIN (G)	3
FAT (G)	12.5
SATURATED FAT (G)	2
CARBOHYDRATE (G)	14

½ cup (55 g) quinoa flakes

1 cup (120 g) almond meal

¼ cup (30 g) gluten-free plain flour

½ cup (140 g) Homemade macadamia nut butter (see page 190)

⅓ cup (115 g) brown rice syrup

1 apple, peeled, cored and coarsely grated

1 teaspoon vanilla extract

¼ cup (45 g) gluten-free chocolate chips or chopped chocolate

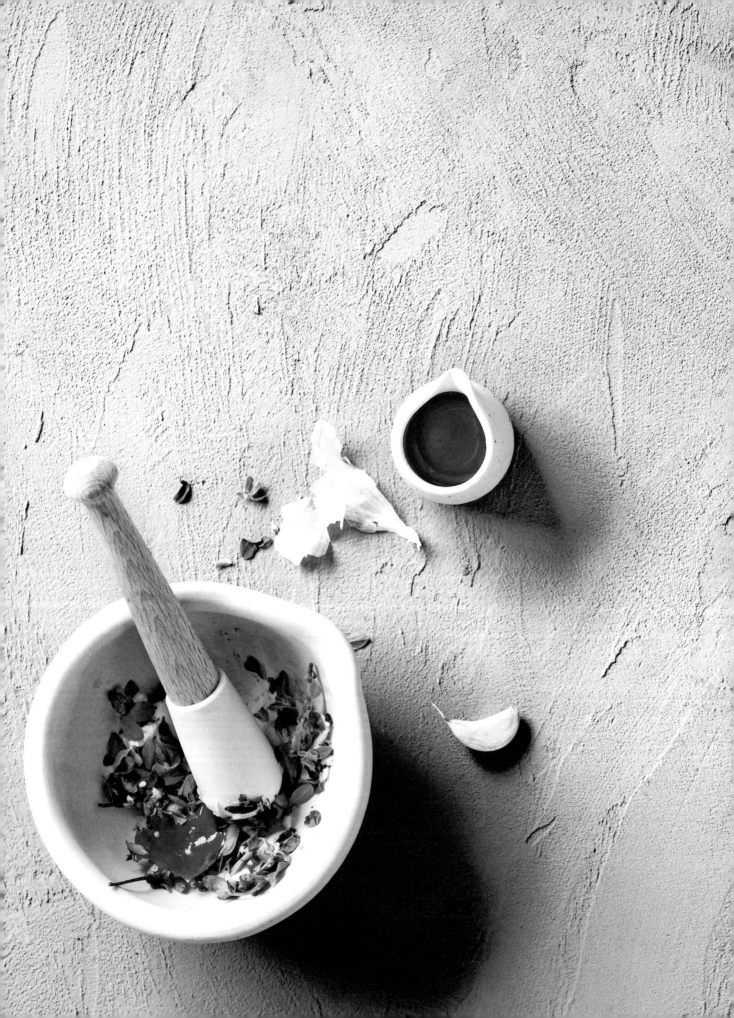

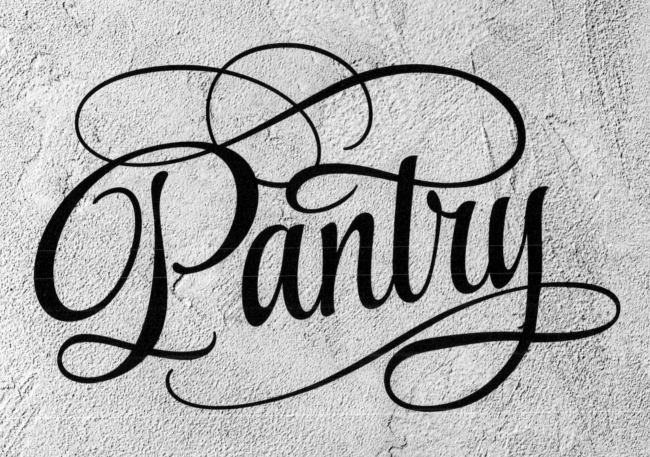

SWEDISH DILL SAUCE

TOBIE This delicious, easy-to-make and, in my mind, essential sauce brings grilled or roasted fish to life. If you don't think you will use it all in one go, it's better to make a half-quantity rather than a large batch that languishes in the fridge.

¼ cup (70 g) gluten-free Dijon mustard

1 tablespoon apple cider vinegar

½ teaspoon sea salt

½ teaspoon cracked black pepper

handful of chopped dill

Put the mustard, vinegar, salt and pepper in a bowl and mix until well combined. Taste and adjust the seasoning, if needed. Fold through the dill and you are ready to go.

TIP This sauce will keep for up to 4 days in an airtight container in the fridge.

SERVES: 6–8

	PER SERVE (FOR 8)
ENERGY (KJ/CAL)	32/4
PROTEIN (G)	0.5
FAT (G)	0
SATURATED FAT (G)	0
CARBOHYDRATE (G)	0.5

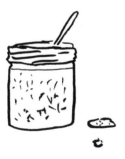

MARJORAM SALMORIGLIO

TOBIE For many years I used fats, such as butter, oils and animal fats like duck fat and pancetta, to flavour foods. And flavour they do, but I've now learned to use herbs and spices instead. Serve this sauce with grilled meats or fish.

2 cloves garlic, halved

pinch of salt

2 small handfuls of marjoram, leaves picked

1 red bird's-eye chilli, chopped

juice of 1 lemon

⅓ cup (80 ml) extra virgin olive oil

cracked black pepper

Put the garlic and salt in a mortar and use the pestle to pound to a paste. Add the marjoram and chilli and lightly pound to combine the ingredients.

Slowly pour the lemon juice onto the paste, while stirring with the pestle to mix it in. Slowly add the olive oil, while stirring with the pestle until the paste loosens up to have a consistency similar to pesto.

Taste the salmoriglio and season with pepper – if you find the flavour a bit too intense, add a little more lemon juice until it is to your liking. (The acidity of the lemon juice will balance the stronger flavours.)

TIP The salmoriglio will keep for up to 2 days in an airtight container in the fridge, but it will be at its absolute best when it's freshly made.

SERVES: 4

	PER SERVE
ENERGY (KJ/CAL)	741/177
PROTEIN (G)	0.5
FAT (G)	18.5
SATURATED FAT (G)	3
CARBOHYDRATE (G)	2

Clockwise from top: Swedish dill sauce, Marjoram salmoriglio and Pickled beets

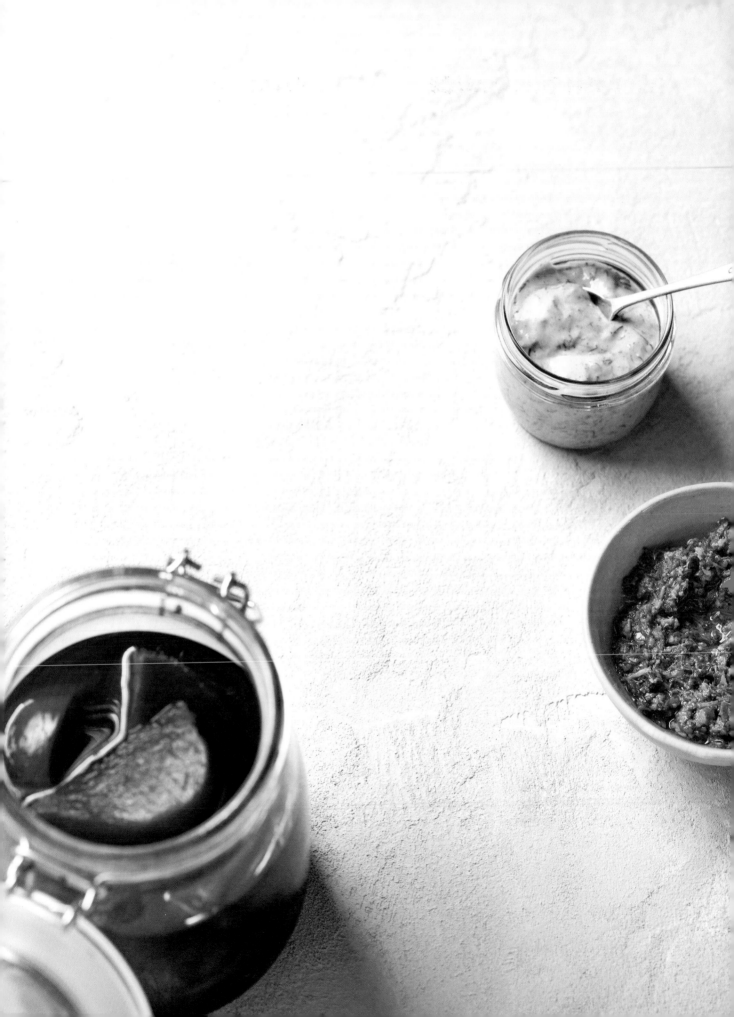

PICKLED BEETS (PICTURED ON PAGE 183)

MAKES: A LOT!

	PER 100 G
ENERGY (KJ/CAL)	297/71
PROTEIN (G)	1
FAT (G)	0
SATURATED FAT (G)	0
CARBOHYDRATE (G)	14

2 kg beetroots of any size, trimmed, leaving about 1 cm of the stalk

2 bay leaves

sea salt

1 litre apple cider vinegar

1 cup (360 g) honey

1 cinnamon stick

2 star anise

¼ teaspoon ground cloves

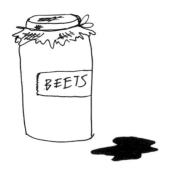

TOBIE I've always loved pickled beets and have been making my own for a while now. I used to use brown sugar as part of the preserving process, but replacing it with honey gives a healthier result and earthier, more natural flavour. The preserving process in this recipe comes from the 2 to 1 ratio of vinegar to water.

GEORGIA Beets are so good for you, and I adore their incredible colour, not to mention flavour. I go through these beets at the rate of knots – Tobie is always wondering why we run out so quickly!

Scrub the beetroots under cold running water, then place in a large saucepan with the bay leaves, a good pinch of salt and enough cold water to cover. Bring to the boil over high heat, then reduce the heat and simmer for about 40 minutes or until a knife can pierce the centre of a beet with ease. When the beets are cooked, drain them in a colander and set aside until cool enough to handle.

Meanwhile, put the vinegar, honey, cinnamon, star anise, cloves, 2 cups (500 ml) water and a good pinch of salt in a saucepan and bring to the boil. Keep the mixture at a rolling boil for 5 minutes.

Wearing gloves to prevent staining, peel away the skin from the beets and take off the tops. Cut the beets into any size you wish – I usually quarter them or cut them into eighths, depending on how big they are. Pack the beets into a hot sterilised jar (see Tips below).

Carefully add the hot brining liquid to the jar, filling it about 2–3 cm from the top. Screw the lid on quite tightly and wipe away any brine from the outside of the jar.

Place a folded tea towel in a deep saucepan large enough to hold the jar, so it covers the base of the pan. Stand the jar upright on the tea towel and fill the pan with water to just above the top of the jar. Bring the water gently to the boil over medium heat, then hold at a boil for 30 minutes. Carefully remove the jar from the pan. Leave to cool.

TIPS Pickled beets will keep for up to 3 months in a cool, dark place. Once opened, store in the fridge.

You'll need a 1.2–1.5 litre capacity sterilised jar, or a few smaller jars, for this recipe. To sterilise the jar, bring a large saucepan of water to the boil. Place the jar in the water so it is fully submerged. Remove after about 5 minutes. Use tongs to transfer the jar to a clean tea towel to drain until it is completely dry. Use as soon as possible.

BASIL PESTO

TOBIE This is a great example of how I have adapted the recipes we eat at home. I've been making pesto for over 20 years and in this version I have simply reduced the quantity of parmesan and replaced some of the extra virgin olive oil with flaxseed oil. In fact, you could replace all of it with flaxseed oil if you want. Note that flaxseed oil needs to be kept in the fridge to prevent it turning rancid and it shouldn't be heated as this destroys its nutritional value.

GEORGIA The important thing to remember here is quantities – if you eat 2 tablespoons of pesto with your dinner, it will end up on your thighs, however 2 teaspoons with your grilled fish is a flavour game-changer. Flaxseed oil, although no less fattening than olive oil, will give you a nice dose of omega 3, which is often deficient in modern western diets.

Toast the pine nuts in a dry, small frying pan over medium heat until golden.

Pop the garlic and pine nuts into a small food processor and pulse until finely chopped. Add the basil and pulse until it is also finely chopped.

With the motor running, slowly pour in the oils. Season with the lemon juice, parmesan, salt and pepper. Pulse to combine, then taste and adjust the seasoning if necessary.

TIP This pesto is best used straight away but will keep in an airtight container in the fridge for up to 1 week.

MAKES: ABOUT ⅔ CUP (150 G)

	PER 35 G
ENERGY (KJ/CAL)	1038/248
PROTEIN (G)	1
FAT (G)	27
SATURATED FAT (G)	3.5
CARBOHYDRATE (G)	0.5

1 heaped tablespoon pine nuts

1 large clove garlic, peeled

50 g basil leaves

50 ml extra virgin olive oil

50 ml flaxseed oil

juice of ½ lemon

1 teaspoon freshly grated parmesan

pinch of sea salt

cracked black pepper

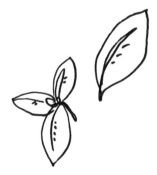

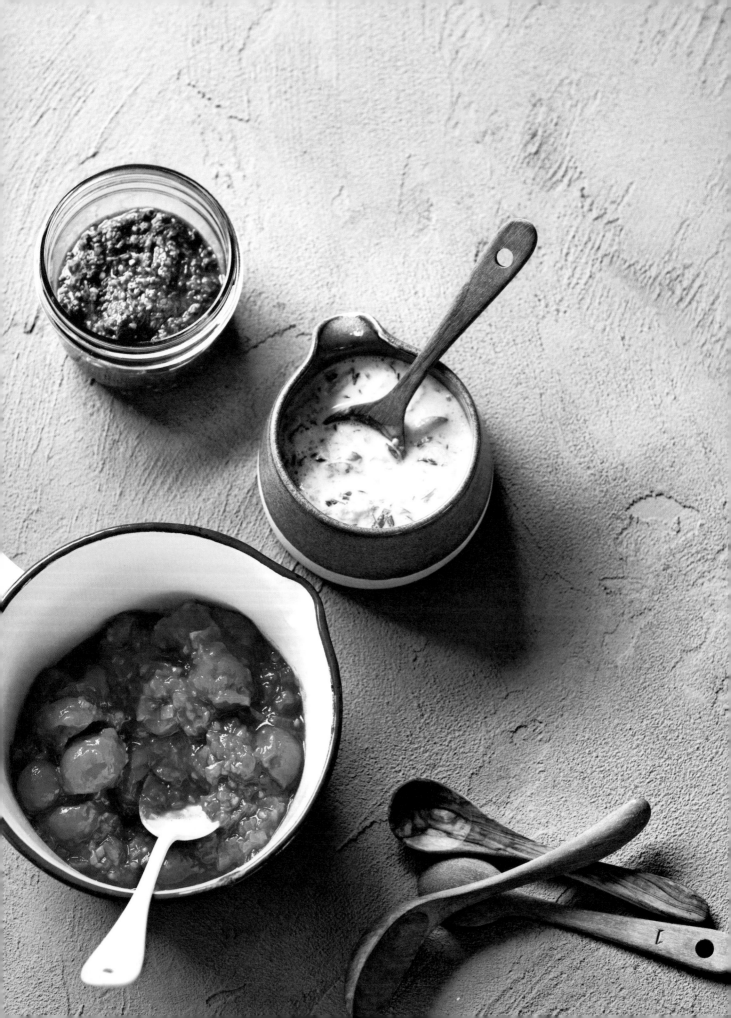

CHERMOULA

TOBIE Chermoula is a spice paste used for meat, fish and sometimes vegetables in Moroccan, Algerian and Tunisian cuisines. The recipe varies from person to person and place to place, sometimes including saffron, onion and various other herbs and spices.

1 bunch coriander, roughly chopped

4 cloves garlic, roughly chopped

5 cm piece ginger, peeled and roughly chopped

1 tablespoon hot paprika

1 tablespoon ground cumin

1 red bird's-eye chilli, roughly chopped

pinch of cayenne pepper

1 teaspoon sea salt

⅓ cup (80 ml) extra virgin olive oil

juice of 1 lemon

Blitz all of the ingredients in a food processor to a thick paste. Use as required.

TIP The chermoula will keep for up to 1 week in an airtight container in the fridge.

MAKES: ABOUT 1 CUP (180 G)

	PER 30 G
ENERGY (KJ/CAL)	514/123
PROTEIN (G)	1.5
FAT (G)	12
SATURATED FAT (G)	2
CARBOHYDRATE (G)	2

NAPOLI SAUCE

TOBIE This sauce makes an excellent base for the pizza on page 130 (there is enough sauce to cover two pizzas). You could also toss it with zucchini (courgette) 'pasta' or serve it with grilled meat, fish or poultry.

1½ tablespoons olive oil

1 small red onion, finely chopped

2 cloves garlic, finely chopped

small handful of basil leaves

400 g tin tomatoes (I use tinned cherry tomatoes)

sea salt and cracked black pepper

Heat the olive oil in a small heavy-based saucepan over low–medium heat. Add the onion, garlic and 2 basil leaves and saute gently for 5–6 minutes, stirring often, until the onion is soft.

Add the tomato, increase the heat to medium–high and bring to the boil, then reduce the heat to low and hold at a very gentle simmer for 15–20 minutes or until the sauce is thick and luscious.

Remove from the heat, season with salt and pepper and fold through the remaining basil leaves.

TIP This sauce will keep for up to 4 days in an airtight container in the fridge.

MAKES: 400 G

	PER 100 G
ENERGY (KJ/CAL)	303/72
PROTEIN (G)	1
FAT (G)	6
SATURATED FAT (G)	1
CARBOHYDRATE (G)	3

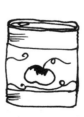

Clockwise from top: Chermoula, Tzatziki and Napoli sauce.

TZATZIKI (PICTURED ON PAGE 186)

SERVES: 4

	PER SERVE
ENERGY (KJ/CAL)	245/59
PROTEIN (G)	4
FAT (G)	1
SATURATED FAT (G)	0.5
CARBOHYDRATE (G)	7

1 Lebanese (short) cucumber, coarsely grated

sea salt and cracked black pepper

200 g low-fat plain Greek-style yoghurt

2 tablespoons finely chopped mint

1 clove garlic, crushed to a paste

TOBIE I've heard it said that tzatziki is the 'dieter's dip', and for good reason – despite it's creamy appearance, there's no guilt trip when you use low-fat plain yoghurt to make it.

GEORGIA I could eat this every day, with anything and everything!

Put the grated cucumber in a fine-meshed sieve over a bowl and sprinkle with a pinch of salt. Set aside for at least 30 minutes to drain off the excess moisture.

Place the salted cucumber, yoghurt, mint and garlic in a bowl and mix to combine. Taste and season with salt and pepper if necessary.

TIP Tzatziki will keep for 2–3 days in an airtight container in the fridge.

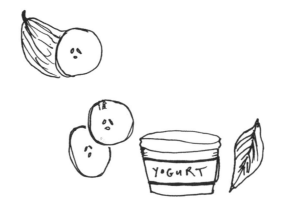

SPLIT ANCHOVY *and* GRILLED LEMON DRESSING

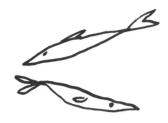

TOBIE I've been using this combination to dress my salads for a while now, but as our diet's improved we have been having it more and more, so it seemed a little crazy not to make larger batches and jar the stuff! I caramelise the lemon here, which drastically changes the flavour of the lemon juice and brings a sweet/sour note to the dressing, but you can use fresh lemon juice instead if you prefer. Note that flaxseed oil needs to be kept in the fridge to prevent it turning rancid and it shouldn't be heated as this destroys its nutritional value.

Heat a grill plate or barbecue until hot. Add the lemon halves, flesh side down, and cook for 5 minutes or until they are starting to char underneath. Remove from the heat and set aside until cool enough to handle. Squeeze the juice into a fine-meshed sieve sitting over a bowl, then use a spoon to scoop out the softened pulp and push as much of it through the sieve as possible.

Put the anchovies, garlic, mustard and lemon juice and pulp in a small food processor and pulse until smooth and well combined. With the motor running, slowly pour in the oils and continue to process until the mixture is well combined. Taste and adjust the seasoning with pepper.

TIP This will keep for up to 2 weeks in an airtight container or jar in the fridge.

MAKES 150 ML

	PER 10 ML
ENERGY (KJ/CAL)	163/39
PROTEIN (G)	0.5
FAT (G)	4
SATURATED FAT (G)	0.5
CARBOHYDRATE (G)	0.5

2 lemons, halved

6 anchovy fillets

1 clove garlic, roughly chopped

2 teaspoons gluten-free Dijon mustard

1½ tablespoons extra virgin olive oil

1½ tablespoons flaxseed oil

cracked black pepper

HOMEMADE MACADAMIA NUT BUTTER

TOBIE I only realised how easy it is to make nut butters quite recently. This version, using macadamias, is totally delicious and you can add other flavourings too if you like, such as cocoa to make an almost Nutella-like spread that goes incredibly well in smoothies. You can use peanuts instead of macadamias if you prefer.

GEORGIA Making your own nut butters is dead easy and so much better for you than buying the commercial varieties. I always make sure we have at least one jar on the go. Note that flaxseed oil needs to be kept in the fridge to prevent it turning rancid and it shouldn't be heated as this destroys its nutritional value.

400 g raw unsalted macadamias	
pinch of sea salt	
1½ teaspoons honey	
1½ tablespoons extra virgin olive oil or flaxseed oil	

Pop the nuts, salt and honey into a food processor and process for 1 minute. Remove the lid and scrape down the sides, then continue to process while slowly adding the oil until the mixture is smooth (this should take about 2 minutes). Transfer to a clean airtight container and store in the fridge.

TIPS The macadamia nut butter will keep for up to 2 months in the fridge.

You can roast the nuts before processing them for a deeper, richer flavour, if you like.

MAKES: ABOUT 400 G

	PER 50 G
ENERGY (KJ/CAL)	1532/367
PROTEIN (G)	3.5
FAT (G)	38
SATURATED FAT (G)	5
CARBOHYDRATE (G)	3

SEED and NUT MIX

TOBIE The way I see it, the trick to maintaining healthy eating is to make the food more-ish and satisfying. For me, texture is a huge part of this and that's where this seed and nut mix comes in. I use this simple recipe at home to sprinkle over dishes like soups, salads, breakfasts, or just to have as a quick snack.

GEORGIA Toasting seeds is something we only started doing quite recently. It gives them a gorgeous nutty flavour and makes them really crunchy. A little sprinkling of this lifts just about anything.

1¼ cups (200 g) pepitas (pumpkin seeds)	
100 g sunflower seed kernels	
100 g slivered or flaked almonds	
100 g pine nuts	

Heat a large heavy-based frying pan over medium heat, add the seeds and nuts and toast gently, moving them around with a wooden spoon so they toast evenly and being careful not to break them, until golden and aromatic.

Remove from the pan and leave to cool completely before storing in a clean airtight container or jar.

TIP Keep in a cool and dark pantry for several months or in the fridge when the weather is warm.

MAKES: 500 G

	PER 25 G
ENERGY (KJ/CAL)	631/151
PROTEIN (G)	5.5
FAT (G)	13.5
SATURATED FAT (G)	1.5
CARBOHYDRATE (G)	2

BLACK OLIVE SAUCE

TOBIE I learnt to make this sauce at The River Café in London, where we served it with roasted or grilled meat and fish. When you're thinking about what to pair it with, bear in mind that the flavour is big so it needs to be able to handle it.

2 big handfuls of black olives, pitted and roughly chopped

2 tablespoons extra virgin olive oil

1 red bird's-eye chilli, finely chopped (optional)

1 clove garlic, finely chopped

cracked black pepper, to taste

1 tablespoon finely chopped marjoram leaves

1 tablespoon finely chopped continental parsley

Put the olives, olive oil, chilli, garlic and pepper in a bowl and stir well to combine. Fold through the herbs and serve right away.

TIP This sauce will keep for 2 days in an airtight container in the fridge. If you like, you can make it without the herbs and it will keep for a couple of weeks – just add the herbs right before serving.

MAKES: 1 CUP (160 G)

	PER 40 G
ENERGY (KJ/CAL)	598/143
PROTEIN (G)	1
FAT (G)	15
SATURATED FAT (G)	2
CARBOHYDRATE (G)	1

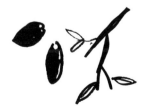

ROAST TOMATO SAUCE

TOBIE This recipe is the wild card in the book – we needed a relish or sauce to accompany another dish on the photo shoot, so I made this and everyone liked it so much that we decided to include the recipe. The intensified flavour that comes from roasting the tomatoes is just beautiful. It's quite rustic and coarse, so using different-coloured tomatoes looks fantastic.

450 g tomatoes (I use a mixture of varieties), cut into wedges if large

1 large clove garlic, unpeeled

1 tablespoon extra virgin olive oil

1 teaspoon thyme leaves

small handful of basil leaves

sea salt and cracked black pepper

Preheat the oven to 200°C and line a baking tray with baking paper.

Spread the tomatoes and garlic clove over the lined tray, drizzle with half the olive oil and sprinkle with the thyme. Roast for 20 minutes or until the tomatoes blister. Set aside for about 5 minutes to cool slightly.

Transfer the tomatoes to a food processor, add the remaining olive oil and tear in the basil leaves. Pulse briefly a couple of times to break the tomatoes up a little. Season to taste with salt and pepper. Use right away or keep in the fridge.

TIP This sauce will keep for up to 3 days in an airtight container in the fridge.

SERVES: 4 (MAKES 600 G)

	PER SERVE
ENERGY (KJ/CAL)	257/61
PROTEIN (G)	1
FAT (G)	4.5
SATURATED FAT (G)	0.5
CARBOHYDRATE (G)	3

MARINATED ROASTED CAPSICUM

1 kg red capsicums (peppers)

½ cup (125 ml) flaxseed oil

¼ cup (60 ml) extra virgin olive oil

¼ cup (60 ml) red wine vinegar

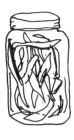

TOBIE This goes with just about anything and we can't get enough of the stuff. There are a few ways you can cook the capsicum – on a hot barbecue, directly over the flame on a gas stovetop, under the oven grill or just in the oven, which is the way I often do it and is probably the easiest method. However you do it, the aim is always the same and that's to blacken the skin, making it easy to remove. You could swap the capsicum for zucchini (courgette), cut lengthways into 1 cm thick strips, or eggplant (aubergine), cut into 1 cm thick rounds. Brush them lightly with olive oil before baking, barbecuing or grilling until tender, then cool before placing in the jars with the oils and vinegar. Note that flaxseed oil needs to be kept in the fridge to prevent it turning rancid and it shouldn't be heated as this destroys its nutritional value.

Preheat the oven to 200°C. Line a baking tray with baking paper.

Place the capsicums on the lined tray and bake for 20 minutes or until the skins are blistered and blackened all over. Remove from the oven and use tongs to immediately transfer to a large heatproof bowl – take care, they will be super-hot. Wrap the bowl very tightly with plastic film and set aside for 15 minutes. The steam from the capsicums will become trapped in the bowl and this helps to loosen the skins from the flesh.

Use your fingers to remove and discard the skin, seeds and cores of the capsicums. Tear the capsicum flesh into strips and set aside until cooled completely. Place the capsicum strips in sterilised jars (see Tips below). Distribute the oils and vinegar among the jars, then screw on the lids quite tightly to seal well. There's no need to let it sit before eating, you can use it straight away if you like. Remove strips of capsicum from the oil mixture as needed, always using a clean utensil to avoid spoilage.

TIPS The capsicum will keep for up to 2 months in the fridge.

You'll need a 1.5–2 litre capacity sterilised jar, or a few smaller jars, for this recipe (see instructions for sterilising jars on page 184).

MUSTARD *and* CAPER MAYONNAISE

TOBIE Mayo is only naughty if you eat too much, too often; a little dollop here and there is nothing but nice. This makes a great accompaniment for roasted or grilled fish.

GEORGIA I'm a massive fan of condiments and always have been, however most of the commercially available ones are loaded with sugar, even the ones that don't taste sweet. This sugar-free mayo tastes great, but use in moderation as always. We're pretty keen on flaxseed oil, which is loaded with omega-3 fatty acids, and it works really well here. Note that flaxseed oil needs to be kept in the fridge to prevent it turning rancid and it shouldn't be heated as this destroys its nutritional value.

Use a balloon whisk to combine the egg yolk and mustard in a large bowl. Slowly add the olive oil or flaxseed oil while gently whisking, until all the oil is added and the mixture is smooth and well combined. Fold through the capers, pepper and vinegar, and serve.

TIPS This mayonnaise will keep, covered with plastic film, for up to 2 days in the fridge.

If the mayo splits while you're adding the oil, put another egg yolk in a clean bowl, then slowly pour the split mayo into the egg yolk while whisking until it comes back together.

SERVES: 4 (MAKES 120 G)

	PER SERVE
ENERGY (KJ/CAL)	912/218
PROTEIN (G)	0.5
FAT (G)	24
SATURATED FAT (G)	4
CARBOHYDRATE (G)	1

1 egg yolk

2 teaspoons gluten-free wholegrain mustard

100 ml extra virgin olive oil or flaxseed oil

2 tablespoons salted baby capers, rinsed and roughly chopped

good pinch of cracked black pepper

2 teaspoons apple cider vinegar

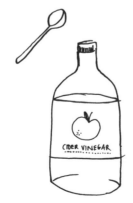

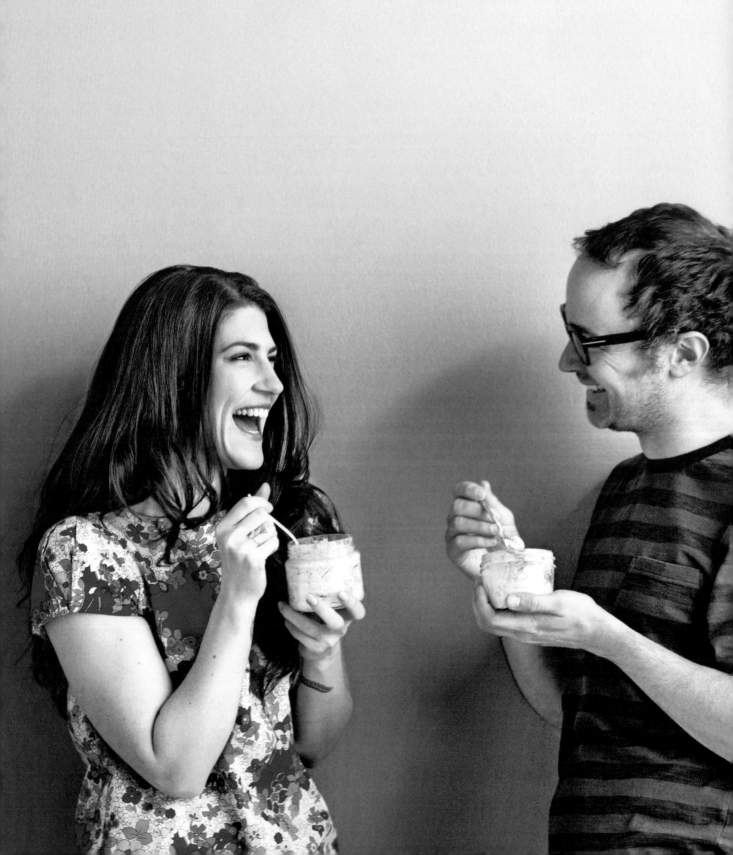

Acknowledgements

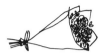

TOBIE This book has been really fun to write and I guess one of the main reasons is that it has had a real purpose for us – Georgia needed to make changes to her diet and that's why we wrote it. So, the first big 'thanks' goes to my beautiful bride and co-author of this book, Georgia Puttock, for pushing my cooking in a totally different direction and giving me the opportunity to learn so much. Also, thank you for hanging out with me (I realise I'm punching above my weight!).

I would also like to thank my mum, dad, sister Lucy and the Katz, Lovett and Barrett families for being the good people they are, and always being supportive through the good, the bad and the ugly. Jamie Oliver, you are a true friend and have shown me that we are only bound by our own thought parameters. Big thanks to Donna Aston, too, for turning my wife into a supermodel.

And another big thanks to all the team at Penguin: Julie Gibbs, who has published my books for almost 10 years and is also a close friend, as well as her amazing team, including Anna Scobie who has worked tirelessly editing this book, Katrina O'Brien, Daniel New and Alissa Dinallo who did the awesome illustrations. Also, thank you to everyone working behind the scenes to make this book happen. You know who you are and if I find you, I'll kiss you on the cheek.

To our sensational shoot team – mega-talented photographer Sharyn Cairns who also shot my last book, *Cook like an Italian*, stylist Lee Blaylock (aka 'Kiwi Jan') and food genius and tall man Andre DeLaine – thank you to you fine people.

And, of course, I wouldn't be able to do what I do without the support of super-agents Justine May, Mim Stacey and Tracy Gualano. I would also like to thank Andrew Freeman and Mei Wu for their amazing support and friendship.

GEORGIA Thank you to my darling husband Tobie. I've taken so much away from you, food-wise, and you've met that challenge with creativity, cheer and support. I must have done something pretty wonderful in a past life to have you in this one.

To my family: Mum, Dad, Nick, Nancy, Matt and especially Tabitha, thank you for your support and belief in me. Thanks also to my friends, especially Monique and Tu-Nu who were my biggest cheerleaders.

Donna Aston: you gave me the ability to change my life. I'm your biggest fan.

AJ, Darren, Chris and Simone: super-trainers, the lot of you. I couldn't have done it without you.

Julie Gibbs and the Penguins: this book is a dream come true, thank you for making it possible.

Sharyn Cairns, Lee Blaylock and Andre DeLaine: I don't think the book could look more beautiful, you guys are superstars.

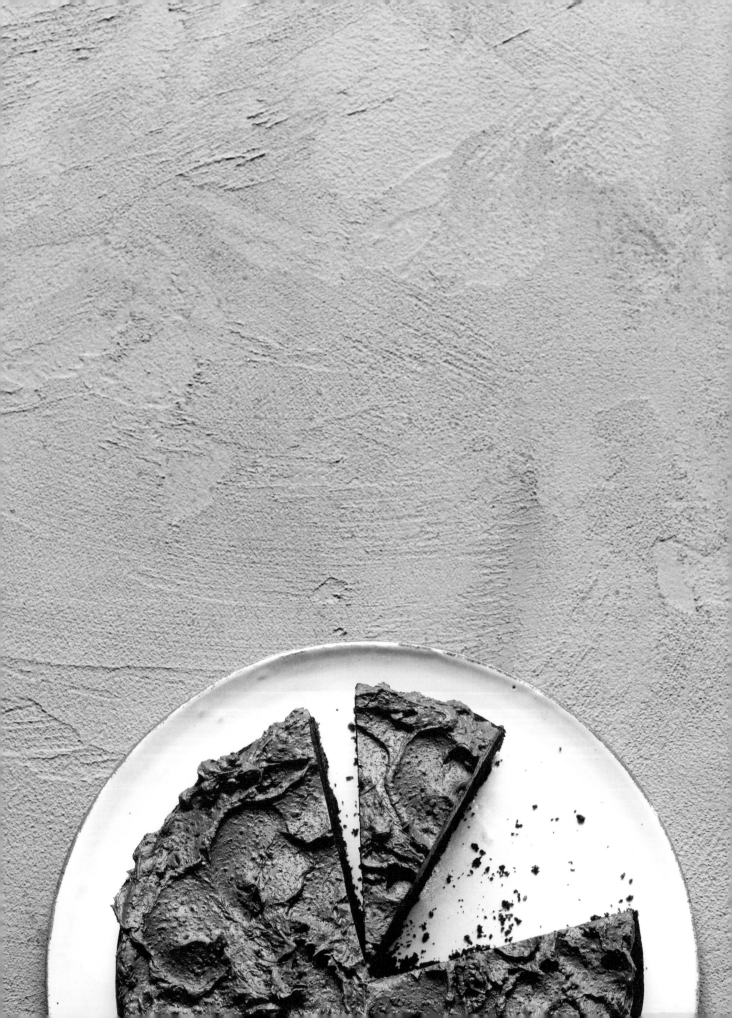

Index

Props

A huge thank you to:
Bettina Willner-Browne
Bridget Bodenham
Brooke Thorn
Bruce Rowe of Anchor Ceramics
Craig Pearce of Urban Cartel
Huset
Kris Coad
Marmoset Found
Safari Living
Sophie Harle of Shiko
Sophie Moran
Wingnut & Co.

LANTERN

UK | USA | Canada | Ireland | Australia
India | New Zealand | South Africa | China

Penguin Books is part of the Penguin Random House group of companies whose addresses can be found at
global.penguinrandomhouse.com.

First published by Penguin Group (Australia), 2015

1 3 5 7 9 10 8 6 4 2

Text copyright © Tobie and Georgia Puttock 2015
Photography copyright © Sharyn Cairns 2015

The moral right of the author has been asserted.

Design by Daniel New © Penguin Group (Australia)
Illustrations by Alissa Dinallo © Penguin Group (Australia)
Photography by Sharyn Cairns
Styling by Lee Blaylock
Typeset by Post Pre-press Group, Brisbane, Queensland
Colour separation by Splitting Image Colour Studio, Clayton, Victoria
Printed and bound in China by 1010 Printing International Limited

National Library of Australia Cataloguing-in-Publication entry
Puttock, Tobie, author
The chef gets healthy / Tobie Puttock
9780670077588 (paperback)
Cooking (Natural foods)
Gluten-free diet--Recipes
Cooking

641.5637

penguin.com.au/lantern